Praise for *Save*

Wow! *Save Yourself from Burnout* is truly a comprehensive and practical manual for both better understanding—but more importantly—reversing job burnout. The expert and experienced authors' view is one I share—that only each of us can ultimately take control of our own physical, mental and emotional health. Sure there are LOTS of doable, highly usable methods in this book (be sure to try out only 2–3 maximum at a time); but as important is how accessible the information and techniques are. This book is both really easy and enjoyable to read. *Save Yourself from Burnout* absolutely stands out for the quality and innovativeness of the methods the authors share as well as for being highly user-friendly in all ways.

    —Robert Pater, Managing Director/Founder, MoveSMART®

Seriously valuable to my life. Thank you.

    —Written attendee comment after workshop at Governor's Occupational Safety & Health Conference, (GOSH) 2017, Portland, Oregon

Save Yourself from Burnout is your one-stop handbook if you're starting to feel stressed out, maxed out, and burned out in your personal or professional life. Written in short, punchy, well-researched chapters, each page is filled with actionable strategies, tactics, and tools to help you become your best self. Marnie and Beth show you how to get your mojo back while boosting your confidence, clarity and control. A total home run. Implement these ideas now and watch how fast your results improve. Bam!!

    —David Newman, author of Do It! Marketing

I'm a firm believer in the old adage "when the student is ready, the teacher will come." Beth Genly and Marnie Loomis are caring and competent teachers, and I wish I had been ready for their insights sooner! Encountering the ideas and engaging in the activities in this book, I feel that I have company on my healing journey, and am not so alone. Instead of a once-through read, this resource will be a valuable companion as I continue to recover from burnout; I anticipate that it will continue to serve me as I practice better habits, so I can avoid going there ever again.

    —Karen Wolfgang, CEO of Independence Gardens

The core challenge in Level III of the Brilliance Game—and a core challenge for too many women at the height of their careers—is to shine as a brilliant star without burning out. This is no easy task. And that's why I ask every Brilliance Game Player to read *Save Yourself from Burnout* and then create her own burnout prevention strategy.

—Tess Daniel, Inventor of the Brilliance Game

Burnout has devastating effects on health and well-being. This book is timely and offers a multitude of customizable solutions for people who are feeling burned out.

—Kelly Campbell, Ph.D., Associate Professor of Psychology, California State University, Santa Barbara; co-host of the radio show "Let's Talk Relationships"

Burnout is more common than you may think. Burnout harms organizations, people and progress. This guide will give you the relief and strategies you need to live a life of confidence and abundance.

—Gary Schmidt, Past International President, Toastmasters International

Hope is a mandatory ingredient for a fulfilling and abundant life. Burnout is the antithesis to this and results in a pervasive loss of this essential element to our health and well-being. Dr Loomis' and Ms Genly's book: *Save Yourself from Burnout* brings hope to all who suffer from burnout. This work also offers hope to all those whom have not yet reached their exhaustive threshold but have begun to slump. In truth, this book is a guide for everyone that wants to reassess, restore, and return to our original birthright—a life filled with anticipation of fulfillment and contentment.

—Erin Lommen, ND, CEO and Associate Medical Director, Labrix Clinical Services, Inc.

Everyone feels the burn when we're close to burning out, but many of us just don't know how to stay productive and joyful. Beth and Marnie show you some very simple and easy to implement strategies for avoiding burnout and building your plan for personal and professional success.

—Cathey Armillas, Marketing Strategist, Speaker and Author of *The Unbreakable Rules of Marketing*

Save Yourself from Burnout

A System to Get Your Life Back

Dr. Marnie Loomis, ND
and
Beth Genly, MSN

Bouclier Press
Forest Grove, Oregon

Bouclier Press
Forest Grove, Oregon
info@burnout-solutions.com
www.saveyourselffromburnout.com

Printed in the United States of America

Design by Jennifer Omner, www.allpublications.com
Back cover photo by Joshua Johnston, joshuajohnstonphotography.com

PUBLISHER'S CATALOGING-IN-PUBLICATION DATA

Names: Loomis, Marnie, author. | Genly, Beth, author. | Rolison, Adam,
  illustrator. | Lawrence, J. A., illustrator.
Title: Save yourself from burnout : a system to get your life back /
  Dr. Marnie Loomis, N.D., [and] Beth Genly, M.S.N. ;
  [illustrated by] Adam Rolison [and] J. A. Lawrence.
Description: Forest Grove, OR : Bouclier Press, 2017. | Includes
  bibliographical references.
Identifiers: ISBN 978-0-9991372-0-8 (pbk.) | ISBN 978-0-9991372-1-5
  (ebook)
Subjects: LCSH: Burn out (Psychology) | Stress (Psychology) | Stress
  management. | Lifestyles—Psychological aspects. | Motivation
  (Psychology) | BISAC: SELF-HELP / Personal Growth / General. |
  SELF-HELP / Self-Management / Stress Management. | HEALTH &
  FITNESS / Healthy Living.
Classification: LCC HD4904.5 .L66 2017 (print) | LCC HD4904.5
  (ebook) | DDC 155.904/2—dc23.

*Dedicated to those too tired to remember
the value they bring to this world.*

Contents

Part I: Learn the Inside Scoop about Burnout

Part II: Create Your Action Plan

Part III: Take Action

Contents

Appendices

List of Interactive Elements

List of Interactive Elements

Preface

In this book, we focus on the things you can do as an individual. We illustrate ways that you can manage burnout risk reduction for yourself, since there is no guarantee that your workplace will change. You'll learn a systematic approach of risk assessment and reduction, ways to increase your resiliency, helpful coping skills to use in your everyday life and strategies to conduct your own continued self-monitoring.

Interactive: You Are Reading the Right Book, If...

Check the statements that apply to your situation.

- ☐ You suspect the line "When the going gets tough, the tough get going," was written for you.
- ☐ You are So. Freaking. Tired.
- ☐ You feel older than your age.
- ☐ You are too busy to spend much time with your family or friends.
- ☐ You are starting to resent your customers or patients.
- ☐ You used to love your career, but the pleasure is gone.
- ☐ You have weeks of unused vacation time, or you lost your vacation time without using it up.
- ☐ You bought a gym membership because they say exercise reduces stress, but you can't remember the last time you went. You have an exercise room, but the equipment has dust on it.
- ☐ You're wondering if you could quit your job and just go be a beach bum for the next 5 years.
- ☐ You've recovered from burnout before, but you're afraid you're going there again.
- ☐ You are concerned that a conversation about burnout with your colleagues, friends or family might result in some type of stigma.
- ☐ You love science-based solutions.
- ☐ Someone gave you this book, saying some version of "Here, I think you need this."
- ☐ You are afraid for a colleague, a friend, or a loved one.

If you checked even one of these, you are reading the right book!

Acknowledgments

Had the two of us not met at a Toastmasters meeting, this book would never have come to be. Not only did the wonderful members of Toastmasters for Speaking Professionals bring us together, they and the members of several other Toastmasters clubs also helped us focus and hone our message and sharpen our speaking skills. Fellow Toastmasters, we are grateful for your constructive criticism, your enthusiasm, and your many challenges that repeatedly took us to the next level. Tom Cox, Susan Bender Phelps, Tara Rolstad, Arlene Siegel Cogen, Allison Hartsoe, James Wantz, Tess Daniel, Jennifer Strait, Phyllis Harmon, Syrena Glade, Karen Wolfgang and everyone else whom we've inadvertently left out of this list: Thank you! Your support continues to mean so much to us.

We feel unbounded gratitude to the pioneering researchers who've dedicated their careers to bringing their curiosity and scientific rigor to answering the questions: "What causes burnout?" and "What helps with recovery and what prevents burnout in the first place?" There are, of course, too many to list them all, but we would like to especially acknowledge Drs. Christina Maslach and Michael Leiter, who have contributed seminal work to this field for decades; your work has inspired and informed ours. In the instances when we refer to specific work done by these many researchers and authors, while we did our best to paraphrase their work faithfully into this book, any errors are, of course, solely our own.

Much appreciation is due to our talented illustrators, J. A. Lawrence, who did the fun "zombie" drawing in the sleep chapter; and Adam Rolison, who drew the Burnout Shield Map, the overloaded donkey and the cortisol graphs.

Many non-Toastmaster friends also encouraged us along the way while we developed our ideas, by critiquing drafts and cheering us up when we thought this book might never be finished. Some names we must mention include: Thea Lopatka, Polly Malby, Dr. Linda Lipstein, Sanne Vallinga, Diane Levin, Robert Pater, Mario Medina. We love you. Thank you for being there for us.

Beth: I am grateful daily for the unfailing support and love I feel from my husband Chris, and my amazing grown children Kim and

Acknowledgments

Caleb; thank you also for your patience and your smart feedback at every stage of this writing process! And to my much-missed parents, Virginia Kidd and James Blish, though neither of them, sadly, lived to read my first book, and to my third parent, much-beloved, very much alive, stepmother Judy Lawrence Blish: you all three vibrantly modeled for me the rewards of delight in the written and spoken word, and instilled the values that guide me daily. All my love!

Marnie: Thank you to the many amazing friends I have been blessed with in this life. To my WF's: Heather, Brookie, Jessica, Kim, Carmin and Amy. To the families of the Traverse City group, my trivia friends, and our FoPo friends. Thank you especially to Cheryl, Katie, Amy and Tony.

Most of all, I'd like to thank my loving family. To my parents, who lead by example and who always freely express their love, excitement and encouragement. To my brother, sister-in-law and extended family members, whom I miss terribly and who make every family get-together a joyous reunion. To my sweetest children: you are the lights of my life! Adena Shea, thank you for your wit and your strength. Luke, thank you for your joy and your courage. Finally, I'd like to thank my love, Peter, for remaining funny and steadfast during stressful times of almost biblical proportions. I'm still a bit surprised we never had locusts.

To everyone we've named and anyone we may have forgotten, thank you for years of kindness, gentleness and encouragement. Neither of us could have gotten out of that deep "hole" of burnout without you.

Part I

Learn the Inside Scoop about Burnout

Chapter ONE

Contrary to Popular Belief,
Burnout Is Not a Workplace Zombie Virus

At a recent teacher's conference, we asked attendees if they saw evidence of burnout in their colleagues. Many of them rolled their eyes at us. "Are you kidding?" they said. "I think pretty much all of us are burned out. It's a huge problem."

Does this sound familiar? Studies show that burnout is a widespread problem in many different professions. Even though so many people experience feelings of burnout, they frequently don't talk about it. Burnout can be very isolating. At the teacher's conference, when asked if they discussed burnout at work, or shared tips for what to do about it, everyone replied, "No, never!" This lack of support often leaves many dedicated, hardworking people who feel burned out wondering, "Am I depressed? Am I a wimp? What is wrong with me?"

One teacher even added, "Some of the people in our school are so obviously burned out, I'm really afraid if I mention it they will just explode and splatter their burnout all over me." That statement really struck a chord with us. Is burnout like some sort of workplace zombie virus?

As goofy as that may sound, we see many parallels. Like a zombie virus, burnout is a condition that is generally feared and not well understood. People worry it could be contagious. Once coworkers have burnout, they keep showing up to work but somehow seem like shells of their former selves. It slows them down and saps their passion and creativity. It usually makes them cranky and can even make them snap at the people around them.

The good news is that no, burnout is not a kind of zombie virus. It is more like a repetitive use injury of the parts of the body that deal with stress. Think more tennis elbow, less *Night of the Living Dead*. In burnout, the brain and endocrine system are affected by certain patterns of long term wear and tear. The body has compensated for so long that it starts to lose efficiency. You can only "red line" your internal engine for so long. Burnout is a medical condition that requires rest and rehabilitation, not zombie quarantine.

Now that we have answers, people can come out of the shadows. People don't need to be afraid any more. While burnout is still out there, there is good information available to help people save themselves and get their old lives back. We are here to help.

Thinking of Burnout as a Type of Injury

Burnout is different than stress. While stress is a state of strain or tension, burnout is the damage that can result from ongoing, nearly unrelieved strain or tension. Burnout is a state in which you act and feel differently, and this different way of acting and feeling happens in very distinct patterns. While stress is a normal and even necessary part of life, it isn't always bad because it isn't always destructive. Many people find stress to be motivating and inspiring. In contrast, burnout drags you down. It consistently makes you less productive and less effective. Stress is a fact of life. Burnout may be common, but it certainly isn't necessary.

Experiencing burnout is different than just having a tough time. It can happen as a result of your workplace stress alone or from a combination of workplace stress and personal stress. Like any other type of injury, the faster you acknowledge your burnout and do something about it, the faster you can get back to feeling normal.

If you have burnout and don't recognize you are injured, you might mistake yourself for being a failure. Consider this scenario: an athlete who doesn't win a race might think of herself as a failure and push herself harder in the next race, but an athlete who doesn't win a race because she is *injured* will focus on recovering from that injury. In sports, injured athletes focus their energy on specific actions for recovery. In life, it is time we take this lesson from the athletes' playbook.

You might be feeling angry with yourself, disappointed, or even ashamed for being burned out. This is quite common; we've spoken with many people who spend a lot of time and energy feeling this way.

Part of this feeling is due to the nature of burnout itself, which can result in feelings of low self-worth (you'll read more about this effect of burnout in Chapter 2.) However, for some of you, these thoughts may be a type of self-talk that you use with the intention to motivate yourself, push harder and succeed. In the past, this may have been a successful strategy for you, but when you are burned out, this kind of thinking only makes things worse.

The difference is that when you are burned out, pushing yourself and expecting to be able to power through won't work—because it can't work. **You are injured.** If you were that runner, would you run the next race without doing anything about your injury? If you did, what would you expect to happen? Running on an injured leg would probably hurt it even more, right? Even if you could somehow manage to win the next race, continuing to run on an injured leg could cause long-term injuries that might end your athletic career for good. The same logic applies to burnout.

Let's take it one step further. If you were the coach for Olympic gold medalist Usain Bolt, would you encourage him to run with an injured leg? Probably not. The benefit of winning one more race is not worth the long-term risk of losing his ability to continue in his overall career. Why should your health and the risk to your career matter any less to you?

Some ways in which burnout is similar to other types of injuries:
- Your performance and overall capacity are affected.
- Recovery requires a healing process.
- This healing process takes time.
- Rest is a necessary component of recovery.
- Some of your daily habits will need to change as you recover.
- Specific "exercises" will help rebuild your strength and resiliency.
- If you continue on as if you aren't injured, you could hurt yourself even more.
- It can be difficult to tell the difference between helpful and hurtful activities.
- Nobody feels like they have time to be injured; injuries are seldom convenient.
- The best way to get better is to take the healing process seriously and commit to it.

If you have been the type of go-getter in life who pushes yourself through the tough times, don't worry. First of all, you didn't necessarily do this to yourself. Research has shown that people don't tend to burn out unless they are exposed to particular types of stress. Second, your strength, commitment, and determination will still play a role as you save yourself from burnout. However, now you will need your strength to help you pull away from your work to look honestly at your situation and consider what is and is not working in your life. Your sense of commitment will be needed to help you learn new skills that will help you recover from your burnout and be resilient against it in the future. And your sense of determination will be necessary to help you stick with the recovery process even though it may be completely unlike you to take a break, or even though you may feel completely exhausted and hopeless at times.

You are not alone and you will not be like this forever. You are injured but you can recover. As you go through this process, we encourage you to find your support community, be gentle with yourself, be patient with the process, and be reassured — you aren't the first to fall into the deep pit of despair we call burnout, and you won't be down there for much longer. We are here to help you get your life back.

Remember:
- Burnout is not weakness.
- Burnout is not all in your head.
- You can recover from burnout.
- You are not alone.

Do You Work in a High-Risk Career?

Burnout is probably found in the highest concentrations in the human service professions, otherwise known as the "helper" professions, including nurses and other medical practitioners, teachers, social workers, lawyers, clergy members, police officers and other professions that deal with assisting the public. There are more studies of burnout in the medical field, social work and teaching than in many other fields. Lawyers and clergy have been the subjects of studies as well.

However, because research on burnout in many other fields is expanding every year, we can say with confidence that burnout shows up in most every field of human endeavor. If you'd like some statistics, here they are:

Helper Professions

Doctors. One 2015 survey reported that on a "typical day" 88% of doctors admit to being "moderately to severely stressed and/or burned out." Most studies show more like 30% to 65% of physicians (depending on specialty) suffer from burnout. Other surveys show those percentages keep rising, year over year. The *level* of physician burnout is increasing as well: in 2015, 66% of physicians felt more stressed / burned out than in 2011.

Nurses. About one-third of all nurses feel burned out.

Mental health workers. 21% to 67% may be experiencing high levels of burnout, with community social workers at highest risk, compared to nurses and psychiatrists.

Teachers. One study in the early 1990's reported 5% to 20% of all American teachers are burned out (depending on the method of assessment.) In 2009, another study found 41% of the teachers (in this admittedly small study) were burned out.

Parish-based clergy. Burnout prevalence rates vary: three different reports gave clergy a burnout rate of 18% to 46%. Even the lowest rate suggests nearly one in five clergy who serve the public are struggling with burnout.

Other Professionals

A sample of 154 **mining accident investigators** averaged a "moderate" level of burnout. (The authors emphasized that we should not confuse a "moderate" burnout score with a "middling" level of burnout; such a score is in fact more severe than just "middling.")

Law enforcement officers. Answering on a specialized burnout scale created for their profession, where a score of 5 indicated the highest level of burnout, law enforcement officers averaged a score of 4.35 in agencies serving towns of less than 100,000 people. Interestingly, burnout appeared to be somewhat less intense for officers in agencies serving more than 250,000 people: they averaged a score of 3.80.

Customer Service

Medical front office staff workers. One survey showed 68% suffer from burnout.

Front line hotel workers. A study showed 15% scored moderate or high levels for burnout.

Hotel middle-managers saw a 32% increase in burnout prevalence between 1989 and 1999. (We feel more recent data on this field of work would be very welcome!)

Grocery workers. A study of frontline grocery workers (such as baggers and shelf-stockers) showed burnout was the *principal* reason for high turnover in this industry. The study authors felt the results of this study suggest that simple efforts to provide motivational slogans or improve low wage structures might not be targeting the real basis of high turnover.

Knowledge Workers

Office Workers. Overall, one survey found 40% of office workers feel burned out. Another study, looking specifically at information technology **(IT) professionals**, found a shocking 100% of this group felt "low personal efficacy" (the third dimension of burnout, as we will discuss in Chapter 2.)

Bankers and financial services workers. 48% reported being "partially" burned out, 13% reported "total" burnout.

Newspaper Journalists. One fairly recent study for this industry found "burnout on the rise." The most at-risk appear to be young copy editors or page designers working at small newspapers.

The Solution to Burnout is a Strategy, Not a One-Time Fix

If we view professional burnout as an injury, and more specifically, a type of workplace injury, then the solution becomes clear. What's the standard response to a workplace injury? It is usually a two-fold strategy. First, the employee's injuries are addressed and treated. Second, an incident report or safety evaluation help to determine how that injury could be avoided in the future. Your own burnout solution can look very much like this strategy. Address your own immediate needs, get your strength and productivity back and then create a plan to avoid burnout in the future. Your burnout may be different than your coworker's, so tailor the steps to your individual needs. Helpful tips or one-time fixes won't likely solve your problem for very long if you ignore your high risk of getting burned out again.

In this book, we focus on the things you can do as an individual. There are other writings focus on the organizational approach to reducing burnout, but this book illustrates ways that you can manage this burnout risk reduction for yourself, since there is no guarantee that your workplace will change. You'll learn a simple but systematic approach of risk assessment and reduction, ways to increase your resiliency, helpful coping skills and habits to use in your everyday life, and strategies to conduct your own continued self-monitoring.

Beyond the Individual: the Business Costs of Burnout

There is a financial incentive for employers to be supportive of their employee's efforts to deal with burnout. Stress and burnout are the source of huge costs to businesses. In 1987, a still widely-used management textbook estimated that American businesses collectively lose $300 billion each year to stress and burnout. In a 2013 report, EU-OSHA updated global estimated losses by region, which increased the US estimate to a collective business loss of $402 billion each year. Yeah, that's billion with a B.

Where does all this financial business loss come from? Decreased productivity is perhaps the most obvious way that burnout is costly. There are many others:

- Decreased productivity
- Staff turnover
- Dysfunctional interpersonal behavior
- Poor customer service
- Absenteeism
- Presenteeism (working while sick)
- Sick leave
- Errors
- Accidents
- Injuries
- Rises in health insurance premiums
- Legal costs
- Disability
- Workplace violence
- Depression
- Alcoholism and drug abuse
- Sadly, even suicide can sometimes be traced to burnout.

Addressing these business and personal "symptoms" individually, while failing to acknowledge burnout as a potential root cause of all of them, can lead to additional costs in wasted effort and misplaced focus. It is time to unmask burnout and face it square-on.

Interactive: The Anti-Burnout Mindset

Are you in the right mindset to save yourself from burnout? Ask yourself: **What are you giving yourself permission to do?** Listen to your answers — you may be surprised.

- ☐ Are you reluctant to give yourself permission to slow down or take a break?
- ☐ Are you expecting more from yourself than you would from anyone else in the same situation?
- ☐ Are you feeling guilty or embarrassed about being burned out in the first place?
- ☐ Would your answers be different if your injury (burnout) was the result of a more conventional injury, like a broken bone?

Just so you know, we used to have these thoughts too! They seem to be common in people who are burned out. In fact, thoughts like these can be a product of burnout itself.

If you do have these thoughts, acknowledge them, but please don't judge yourself. Recognize them for what they are. Pushing or motivating yourself with these kinds of thoughts may have been a coping mechanism that helped you through tough times in the past. As a result, thinking this way may have become a habit. In order to break that habit, you'll need to recognize when it happens. Then you can start the process of forming a new, healthier mindset.

Reassure yourself that by taking the time and effort to recover from burnout, you are doing what is necessary to heal. You will be getting your life back, and by doing so, you'll be much more productive in the future. Also, when you save yourself from burnout, you'll be helping the people around you as well.

Message of Hope

It is time to end the silence around burnout with a message of hope: **Burnout can be beaten.** Burnout research conducted over the last few decades has helped to demystify burnout, uncover causes and identify solutions. Our intention for this book is to compile all this helpful information into an easy-to-use system for doing something about it.

We are two burned-out healthcare providers who developed this system as part of a very personal quest to deal with our own burnout. We know how much you need this information and how little energy you have to spend on it. The recovery process is gradual but possible. Your future self will thank you. **You are worth it.**

Questions

← —— Cosmo type Quiz.

I was a burnout Socual Worker, & Educator who is committed to helping others thru e work.

☐ Do you feur

Chapter TWO

How Does Burnout Happen?

Burnout is a consequence of a person's prolonged attempts to protect themselves from emotional and interpersonal stressors. It is characterized by three main dimensions: the feeling of **emotional exhaustion** (which includes physical and mental exhaustion), a sense of **cynicism** (feeling less caring about the people you work with; older studies use the word *depersonalization* for this dimension,) and a **low sense of personal accomplishment** (feeling like you can't be effective or your work doesn't matter). Within the medical research, there are a few other definitions floating around. In this book, we use the definition above, which is based on work by the scientist, Christina Maslach, PhD, who developed the widely used measurement of burnout, the Maslach Burnout Inventory.

How It Happens: The Big Picture

From a big picture perspective, the process of burnout stems from chronic stress and a person's response to that stress over time. The big picture of burnout also extends into your social relationships as well. In fact, in a 2016 article, Maslach and Leiter say, "The significance of this three-dimensional model is that it clearly places the individual stress experience within a social context and involves the person's conception of both self and others."

Research has found that certain types of stress are more likely to cause burnout than others. Burnout isn't a problem of "weak" or flawed people. Burnout is the result of a combination of external and internal factors, and therefore, there will be more than one strategy you can use for reducing your burnout risks.

If you are in a high-risk environment, you can avoid burnout by either getting out of that high-risk environment or by being aware of and changing your reactions to stress and increasing your internal protective factors. A good metaphor for avoiding emotional burnout from stress is avoiding getting burned by fire.

Consider how fire, in one form or another, needs to play a role in our everyday lives, just like stress does. We cook with fire, we heat our homes with it, we power our vehicles with it. In general, if you don't want to get burned, you keep your distance from it. However, if you have to work near fire in any capacity, say as a cook or even a firefighter, then you maximize your protection against it. You continually keep track of your environmental risk and you make safety a primary goal.

This expectation that firefighters will put a high priority on safety and risk awareness is standard within the firefighting industry. Hopefully, as we come to have a greater understanding of burnout risks in the general work environment, avoiding emotional burnout will become the industry standard for those in business as well.

The Camel and the Straw

You are probably familiar with the saying "The straw that broke the camel's back." It demonstrates how, when tensions have been building, one small thing can set off a catastrophic event.

Before the breaking point, changes can still be made. After that point, the damage is more difficult to repair (for the unfortunate camel, perhaps impossible.) Dealing with burnout is similar in many ways. How can you tell when you are getting close to your breaking point? And also, which is the better strategy, prevention or repair?

Think about all the important factors at play in the years, weeks and days leading up to that poor camel's back being broken. Was the straw loaded properly? Had the camel been carrying unusually heavy loads in the recent past? How healthy was the camel? Had it slept or eaten lately? Was it being cared for properly?

Humans and their responsibilities are far more complicated than camels and straw. Yet the metaphor is still useful when considering how burnout happens and how to prevent it. In both situations, many factors affect whether the one doing the work will be able to survive under the pressure. Both sides matter: the stress of the burden and the one carrying it.

Factors that Lead to Burnout: The Straw

What are the external factors that lead to burnout? Research has shown that in the workplace, there are six types of stressful situations most likely to lead to burnout. As identified by Christina Maslach and Michael Leiter, stress caused by one or more of these six "mismatches" between you and your work environment has been found to significantly increase your risk for burnout.

- A sense of control
- Receiving sufficient reward
- Having a sense of community with your colleagues
- Feeling you are being treated fairly
- Feeling that your core values are shared by the organization
- Feeling that you have a reasonable workload with the necessary resources to complete it.

To give an idea of how Drs. Maslach and Leiter assess potential sources of burnout, here are a few items from their book, *"Banishing Burnout: Six Strategies for Improving Your Relationship with Work."* Please note, however: they emphasize that this is not a complete survey.

For each item, think about how your current work matches up with your personal preferences, work patterns, and aspirations.

	Just Right	Mismatch	Major Mismatch
Workload			
The amount of work to complete in a day			
The frequency of surprising, unexpected events			
Control			
My participation in decisions that affect my work			
The quality of leadership from upper management			

	Just Right	Mismatch	Major Mismatch
Reward			
Recognition for achievements from my supervisor			
Opportunities for bonuses or raises			
Community			
The frequency of supportive interactions at work			
The closeness of personal friendships at work			
Fairness			
Management's dedication to giving everyone equal consideration			
Clear and open procedures for allocating rewards and promotions			
Values			
The potential of my work to contribute to the larger community			
My confidence that the organization's mission is meaningful			

Table 2.1 Quick assessment of six areas of worklife (used by permission)

- If everything is a match, you have found an excellent setting for your work.
- A few mismatches are not very surprising. People are usually willing and able to tolerate them.
- A lot of mismatches, and especially major mismatches in areas that are very important to you, are signs of a potentially intolerable situation.

Outside of the workplace, stress from other sources can contribute to your burnout as well. For instance, social support, financial stability, housing security, emotional trauma from illness or death of a loved one, divorce, personal injury or illness, or legal troubles can all play a role. Even otherwise happy occasions, such as getting married or participating in major holidays, can create significant stress that adds to the growing pile of "straw." We go over these more specifically in Chapter 5, where we show how these factors fall into five different groups and how to keep track of your status in each of them.

These **Five Key Areas** of your Burnout Shield, as we call them, are your:
- Level of **Self-Care**
- Practices of **Reflection & Recognition**
- Functional **Capacity** based on who you are, how your life is structured and how much you have on your plate
- Involvement in your **Community**
- **Coping Styles** you use

Factors That Lead to Burnout: The Camel

The other part of that metaphor, the camel, refers to the one bearing the load. What about you could make you more susceptible to burnout? Several kinds of things can add to your vulnerability, such as aspects of your personality and temperament, your habits, coping methods and physical health. The changes that happen in the body while you've been responding to long-term stress can also affect your physical health and make you more susceptible to burnout.

"What the Heck Is Wrong with Me?"

One of our favorite audience reactions is the look of relief when they realize that their symptoms of fatigue, irritability and low sense of personal accomplishment could all be due to burnout. Up until that point, almost all of them have told us they were wondering, "What the heck is wrong with me?"

If burnout were as simple as something that was all in your mind, like a bad attitude or a flawed type of thought pattern, perhaps it would be simple to stop that thought pattern and instantly recover. But burnout is more complicated than that. Chronic stress can have a negative impact on the body. In order to save yourself from burnout, you also have to address your physical needs.

How Chronic Stress Affects Your Body

When it comes to reacting to a stressful situation, the mind and body are very closely connected; the body is hard-wired to quickly and fiercely respond. This makes sense for dangerous situations where you need to respond quickly in order to save yourself. However, the body pretty much responds the same way to all types of stress. It isn't wired to deal with life-irritating stress in a different way than life-threatening stress. Therefore, responding to chronic stress takes a toll on your body. Here are some of the main issues:

General.
- Lowered immunity resulting in more frequent illness and infection.
- Changes in food cravings.
- Field of vision narrows.
- Weight gain (especially around the waist and hips.)
- Increased sensitivity to light, smell or noises.

Muscles. Your muscles act like a system of pulleys, they are designed to tense up and relax, tense up and relax. This way they allow you to move and maintain your posture. However, when under chronic stress, you experience:
- Muscles that are constantly tense, which can negatively affect your posture and make it more difficult to move properly.
- Your body in a constant state of being "guarded."
- Tension-type headaches
- Migraines
- Chronic pain conditions (these are more common in someone who has an injury during a time that they have also been experiencing chronic stress.)

Nervous System. The nerve control of your body's physical response to stress is directed by your autonomic nervous system (ANS). This system operates by balancing two different settings: the sympathetic (SNS) and parasympathetic (PNS) settings. Only one of these settings is the dominant one at any given time.

The sympathetic (SNS) setting is known as your "fight or flight" response. This is your body's emergency mode. This shifts all of your body's resources to the parts needed to fight or run away from something that might kill you. If your body could yell, "BATTLE STA-TIONS, BATTLE STATIONS, ALL HANDS ON DECK!" and tell the cooks and the laundry guys and the plumbers to all drop what they were doing, ignore their usual jobs and grab a weapon, it would happen while it was in the SNS setting.

The other setting, the parasympathetic (PNS) setting, doesn't have a nickname, but if it did it would be your "keeping your body operating efficiently" response. This is your normal functioning mode. The PNS shifts your body's resources to the parts of the body that take care of normal business like digesting food, making repairs, and getting rid of waste. For long-term health, your body is designed to have the PNS setting as the dominant setting, with brief interruptions by the SNS setting.

- When you are chronically stressed, the body stays in the sympathetic (SNS) "fight or flight" mode for extended periods of time. This does not allow your body to efficiently perform day-to-day activities such as digest food, get rid of waste or conduct repairs.
- When the SNS is dominant, it signals your adrenal glands to release the hormones adrenaline and cortisol. These endocrine hormones rapidly spread the panic signal throughout your body and cause your heart to beat faster, your breathing rate to increase, your blood sugar levels to increase and your circulation to shift from your internal organs out to your arms and legs.

Mental/Emotional.

- Distraction, resulting in higher rates of error and injury.
- Depression
- Anxiety/Fantasizing about illness or injury (as a mental way to escape a situation that seems otherwise inescapable.)

Heart and Circulation.

- Repeated stress on the heart and blood vessels which can lead to long-term problems.
- Increased inflammation, especially in the coronary arteries, which can increase your chance of heart attack.
- Hypertension (high blood pressure)
- Heart attack
- Stroke

Breathing. Chronic stress causes your breathing to be more shallow and rapid, which:
- Can bring on a panic attack in someone prone to them.
- Can make it more difficult to breathe for people with breathing disorders.

Gastrointestinal. Chronic stress can cause problems all along your digestive system.

In your esophagus, it can cause:
- Acid reflux (heartburn.)
- Changes in eating patterns (eating more or less than usual.)

In your stomach, stress can cause:
- An increased awareness of the sensations in your stomach (feelings of "butterflies.")
- Vomiting
- Nausea
- Stomach pain
- Ulcers

In your intestines, stress can cause:
- Decreased blood flow to the intestines resulting in less efficient digestion and absorption.
- Diarrhea
- Constipation

Endocrine. The stress signals triggered by your body being in sympathetic (SNS), or "fight of flight" mode signal two main areas to respond:
- Initially, chronic stress will lead the adrenal glands to produce cortisol and epinephrine.
- After long-term chronic stress, the adrenal gland may not be able to produce adequate amounts of cortisol and levels can become abnormally low throughout the day, leaving the person to feel exhausted all day long. These consistently low cortisol levels can also disrupt the sleep/wake cycle.
- Cortisol and epinephrine stimulate the liver to produce more glucose, a blood sugar that gives the body a burst of energy. For

people who have a high risk of blood sugar problems, this can increase their risk of diabetes.

Chronic stress can also affect *sexual desire, performance and reproduction:*
- Decreased sexual desire
- Issues with sexual performance
- Fertility issues due to effect of chronic stress on the balance of hormones

In women, the impact of chronic stress on hormone balance can impact their menstruation:
- Stress can cause irregular or even missed menstrual cycles.

  Stress can caused prolonged or heavier menstrual bleeding. This is due to the body's ability to convert progesterone into cortisol during times of extreme stress. Unfortunately, this increased loss of blood can lead to anemia, which makes people feel exhausted and foggy-headed, which often leads to more stress.
- PMS symptoms such as cramping, fluid retention, bloating, negative mood and mood swings can all be more intense when a woman is under chronic stress.
- The symptoms of menopause, such as hot flashes, mood changes, anxiety and feelings of distress can be an additional form of stress, which can become overwhelming if the woman is already experiencing chronic stress
- Chronic stress can cause more frequent or intense hot flashes

In men, the impact of chronic stress on hormone levels can have many effects on their bodies:
- Interruptions in the reproductive system and development of healthy sperm
- Decreased sperm counts
- Erectile dysfunction
- Impotence
- Decreased testosterone production:
  - Low testosterone can result in fatigue, irritability.
  - Low testosterone has also been linked to higher rates of metabolic syndrome and diabetes.

Beyond Chronic Stress: Burnout Can Affect Your Body

Burnout is a hot topic in medical research, so new information is constantly being discovered about how exactly burnout happens and how it affects the body. With what we know already, there is enough information to fill an entire book with related medical issues. For the purposes of this book, we will cover some of the big picture aspects. These pieces of information have given us the biggest "Aha!" moments as we've tried to understand our own reactions during burnout and have helped our audiences and patients the most as well. Hopefully for those of you who have been getting really disappointed with yourselves, this will also help you start to see that there are actual physical reasons you have been feeling the way you do. Hopefully you can forgive yourself and move on to the next stage, healing.

How Burnout Can Make Your Brain Work Differently

Certain brain scans can show which part of the brain is active when people participate in different activities. When scientists do scans on burned-out people as they work, and compare them to the brains of non-burned out people as they work, it shows that burned out brains are active in different areas than non-burned out ones. During the process of becoming burned out, you have inadvertently trained yourself to use a different, less effective part of your brain to deal with incoming information and solve problems. The good news is that you can train it back!

Even though you may not realize it, when you take part in repetitive activities, especially ones that are linked to good or bad feelings, you are changing your brain and training it. The saying in neurobiology, "You wire what you fire," refers to the way the brain is constantly changing over time, depending on how you use it. If you use a particular pathway frequently, your body builds up more neurons in that area to support that particular function.

Visualize your brain as having two networks, the Reactive part and the Reflective part. These two networks in the brain both process incoming information and work on problem solving, but they do it in different ways. Your body chooses one of these to act as your brain's default setting, so there is always one or the other, either the Reactive part of the Reflective part, that is standing by, ready to handle the information coming in and the problems that are waiting to be solved.

The Reactive network is the less evolved part of your brain. This is the network in your brain that reacts with involuntary behaviors and emotions without the chance for you to consciously think about them first. When you process incoming information with this part of your brain, you experience lower endurance and feel pain more intensely and for longer periods of time. Also, when you use this part of your brain to solve problems, you are less creative and tend to act impulsively.

In comparison, the Reflective network of your brain is the more evolved part. This is the network in your brain that reacts in a careful, thoughtful manner. When you are using this part of your brain, any pain that you feel is experienced as being less intense and lasts for a shorter time. Also when you use this part of your brain to solve problems, you have more control over your emotions, you are able to reason, and you have a greater ability for creative problem solving.

So if you have been in a long-term situation where you have experienced chronic stress and your efforts don't often get met with any sense of success or reward, your brain can become trained to equate effort with failure. This repetitive action trains your brain to use the Reactive network. The good news is that you can train it back into the Reflective mode! You can reset this mode by exercising your brain using techniques we discuss in Chapter 7.

How Burnout Can Affect Your Internal Clock
(affecting metabolism, sleep/wake, immunity, brain function, and heart function)

As you probably know, your adrenal glands help you deal with stress. However, the adrenal glands are not used only for stress responses. They are also part of the complicated system that feeds into your sophisticated internal master clock. This internal master clock coordinates the timing and function of your sleep/wake cycle, metabolism, immunity, brain function and cardiovascular system. By sending you cues for important functions like when to sleep, when to wake, and when to get hungry, this internal clock helps you to anticipate and be ready for the typical parts of your day. As you can imagine, if you are under chronic stress and the function of your adrenal glands gets thrown off by an excessive need to respond to it, your entire master clock can get out of whack.

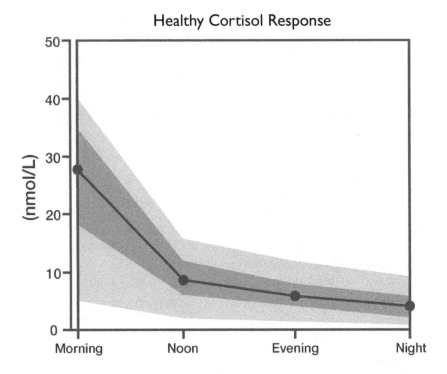

Your doctor can actually test to see how your adrenal glands are doing. Are they functioning correctly as part of your internal master clock? This test, which looks at your diurnal (during the day) salivary cortisol levels, measures cortisol at four times throughout the day.

When you are healthy, your highest cortisol level happens in the morning and will gradually decrease to the lowest levels in the evening. The early morning spike in your cortisol level is what signals your body to wake in the morning.

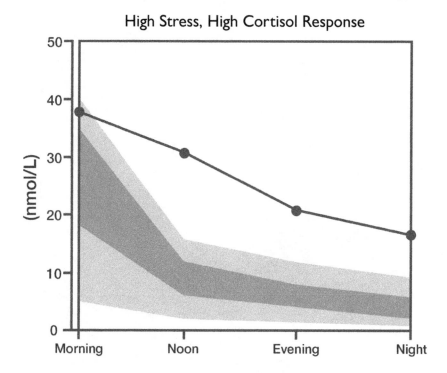

High Stress, High Cortisol Response

If you have been responding to fairly severe stress and are relatively early in your process of chronic stress response, your cortisol levels will be high at several times throughout the day.

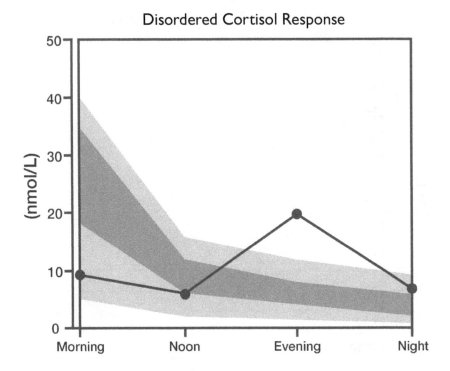

Disordered Cortisol Response

If your sleep/wake cycle is off because you keep odd hours or have a chronic lack of sleep, your cortisol spike might happen in mid-afternoon (or later,) when it isn't supposed to. As you can imagine, it is difficult for people with a late cortisol spike to get to sleep at night, since their body's internal clock is telling them to wake up.

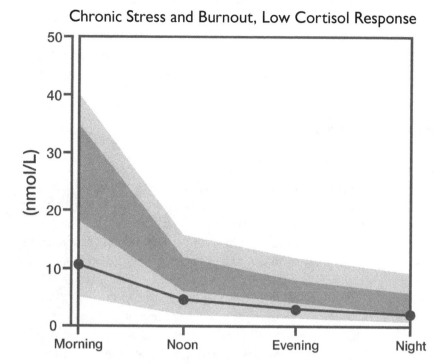

Chronic Stress and Burnout, Low Cortisol Response

And finally, if your adrenal glands aren't able to function for any reason, which includes being worn out from a long-term chronic stress response, your diurnal cortisol levels can be much lower in the morning or even fairly flat all day. When this happens, you feel exhausted all day.

Lab studies have shown that consistently low diurnal cortisol levels throughout the day tend to be found in people experiencing that third dimension of burnout, (exhaustion, a sense of cynicism, **low sense of personal accomplishment**).

Paying attention to cortisol levels is important for a couple of reasons. First of all, a healthcare practitioner familiar with these issues can prescribe therapies to support your adrenal function. There are several important nutrients, botanical medicines and even hormonal therapies that can help to rehabilitate your adrenal glands and gently support normal function.

Second, if you've been feeling depressed and you aren't sure if you are "just" depressed or if your depression is part of your burnout, understanding the role of burnout can help your doctor know where to start. This is important, because if you have only depression, your doctor should treat the depression, but if you have depression as part of burnout, your doctor should treat your burnout first, because the treatment for depression may make your burnout, and your depression, worse.

The Burnout Solution

Who or What Needs to Change?

If burnout is a problem, which one needs to change, you or your organization? That's the tricky part. The better question might be "Which one *can* change?" or more importantly, "Which one do *you* have the power to change?" The place where you have the most power is with yourself, so in this book, we focus on you and your resiliency. The skills we cover here will serve you no matter what type of work environment you find yourself in.

On the one hand, research suggests that thoughtful, targeted organizational change can have the biggest potential to reduce employee burnout. On the other hand, you may not be able to wait for that process. Anything on an organizational level may be completely out of your control. Even if you could start that process, that may not be the best way to approach your own recovery. If you are burned out, issues like budgetary constraints, third party regulations, or even the very nature of the work could be creating issues that would be difficult to control or address.

Another benefit of focusing on yourself is that we feel the current studies of burnout may not be addressing some of the more personal factors that aren't largely considered, such as standing up against social or family pressures, expecting to be the representative of an entire cultural/gender group, the need to be strong for the sake of others, etc. We've both had personal family challenges that we wouldn't even consider walking away from, so it was incredibly important that our burnout healing process addressed all of these issues.

Our intention is to provide you with the resources to build a set of skills that will work for your benefit either way. These skills will give you the greatest fighting chance, no matter what your work or home environment is like.

The KISSY Method

We nicknamed our approach the KISSY method: **Keep It Simple, Save Yourself.** With the KISSY method, you save yourself from burnout by making low-effort changes that are completely within your control. Once you've provided some initial relief to yourself and get your strength back, you'll have the energy to reevaluate and figure out what to do next. With the KISSY method, you can be reassured that even the initial precious energy you put forth has a strong chance of coming back to benefit you directly.

It's true that individual changes may not completely save you from burnout. Major workplace factors contribute to your burnout as well. But for those of you who either aren't in a position to change the organization around you, or who simply don't have the time to wait, starting with yourself is a smart option.

One more thought for you go-getters out there: As strong as your urge may be to fix an obvious problem, fight an unjust system or help others before helping yourself, it is crucial to take care of your own immediate needs. Think back on the lesson we all learn every time we fly in a plane. "In the unlikely event that air pressure drops and oxygen masks drop down in front of you, place your mask on yourself before helping others." If you are currently suffering from burnout, you won't be much help to others if you don't help yourself first. You need relief now!

Moving Forward: What to Expect from the Rest of this Book

As you continue to read this book, you will learn how to gently but effectively save yourself from burnout. Conserving your energy is key. If you are burned out, your energy needs to be protected. With every effort you put forth, try to "feed two birds with one seed" as one colleague used to say. That means to try and get as much benefit out of everything you do. We will show you how.

First, we'll help you to **simplify your problem list.** Chances are, you've been feeling like there are so many problems in your life right now, you don't know where to start. Thankfully, many of those problems very likely have the same root cause — burnout! Burnout is one problem that can disguise itself as many different individual ones. For example, if you have been dealing with depression, relationship problems, work performance issues, sleep issues, getting sick all the time, weight gain, crippling self-doubt, and many other serious issues that we cover in Chapter 3, you don't need to exhaust yourself trying to solve all of these different individual problems, you only need to focus on the one central issue: burnout. When your burnout improves, these other problems will improve as well. As you read this book, you'll learn how to spot burnout in its many different forms and recognize all the changes it has caused in your life. Burnout won't be able to fool you anymore.

Second, we'll help you create your **plan of attack.** Learn how to find your burnout strengths and weak spots by taking our individualized **Burnout Shield Self-Tests** in Chapter 5. You'll learn to evaluate the five Key Areas of your life where individual changes can make a difference. You'll identify which of your personal habits are protecting you and which are making you more vulnerable. It may seem like this is common sense stuff, but it isn't always obvious!

Third, depending on the results of your individualized Burnout Shield Self-Tests, you'll learn how to **take effective action** with the KISSY method in each of your five Key Areas where individual changes can help. Learn which options are likely to bring you the most benefit with the least amount of effort. Start with the focus on yourself, get some relief, and when you have regained some of your strength and energy (be gentle with yourself!), then you can look into what can be done to change the work environment around you.

Chapter THREE

Recognizing Burnout When You See It and Feel It

Burnout hurts. When you burn out at work, you feel diminished, like a part of yourself has gone into hiding. Challenges that were formerly manageable feel insurmountable.
—Monique Valcour, MS, PhD

One of the biggest problems with burnout is that people often don't know they have it. They deny it, don't understand it, or think that they have somehow become a bad person. Burnout is a real thing and this chapter introduces some of the ways to verify it.

The Three Dimensions of Burnout

Burnout is not just a bad day, or fatigue after a big project. Burnout can include soul-deep exhaustion withdrawal from work and life activities, and even deep doubts about your own ability to make a difference.

Burnout has three dimensions:

- **Emotional Fatigue.** Feeling overextended or depleted. This dimension also includes physical fatigue, which is often profound.
- **Cynicism.** Losing the feeling of the people around you as humans to whom you are connected. Instead, seeing them more as problems you have to solve, as "others" who are not part of your "tribe," or even as objects in your way. It is marked by a distant attitude toward one's work and the people one works with. Other words that are used for Cynicism include: distancing, disconnection, and withdrawal.

- **Inefficacy.** Another medical word. Inefficacy means you feel your efforts cannot make a difference (even if you used to know your work is highly valuable.)

Harvard HelpGuide has a useful table (used by permission) on the differences between stress and burnout:

Stress vs. Burnout	
Stress	**Burnout**
Characterized by over-engagement	Characterized by disengagement
Emotions are over-reactive	Emotions are blunted
Produces urgency and hyperactivity	Produces helplessness and hopelessness
Loss of energy	Loss of motivation, ideals, and hope
Leads to anxiety disorders	Leads to detachment and depression
Primary damage is physical	Primary damage is emotional
May kill you prematurely	May make life seem not worth living
Harvard HelpGuide's Source for this table: *Stress and Burnout in Ministry.* **(See Appendix C for more information.)**	

Table 3.1 Some "soft" differences between being overstressed and burned out

Interactive: How Burnout Feels

When speaking to a group, we often ask our listeners to talk about how a burned-out person might feel, along each of these dimensions. Our audiences never fail to amaze and move us with the eloquence of their answers. (We never put them personally on the spot, but it does seem pretty likely that many of them are speaking from personal experience with burnout.) Here are a few of their responses:

Emotional Exhaustion: Feeling over-extended and depleted.

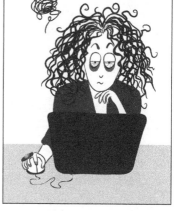

- *Overburdened*
- *Sad*
- *Isolated*
- *Weary*
- *Exhaustion that is "bone-deep," or even "soul-deep"*
- *Nothing seems fun*
- *I used to love my job, but now...*
- _____

Cynicism: Disconnected, distant attitude toward one's work, and the people one works with.

- *Suspicious*
- *Resentful*
- *Critical*
- *Irritable*
- *Cranky*
- *Snappish*
- *Disconnected*
- *Withdrawn*
- *Lonely*
- _____

Inefficacy: Loss of the sense that your efforts can make a difference.

- *Inertia*
- *Just can't climb that wall again*
- *Apathetic*
- *Feel like a fraud*
- *Afraid to let the professional veneer slip*
- _____

Now it is your turn. Which ones resonate for you? What words would you put on your list of how burnout feels to you?

Are You Burned Out? How to Tell

Here we'll discuss two of the research-tested ways to evaluate yourself for burnout: the official MBI test and the short self-test. According to the research on burnout, they work about equally well.

Maslach Burnout Inventory (MBI,) the most commonly accepted test. Most of the initial heavy lifting in burnout research was done (and is still being done) by Christina Maslach, PhD. She created a psychological assessment tool, a questionnaire now called the Maslach Burnout Inventory, or MBI. The MBI, while not in the public domain, is widely used in burnout research and can be taken by individuals. The MBI includes multiple questions on all three of the burnout dimensions, emotional exhaustion, cynicism and inefficacy.

If you want to purchase the right to administer the MBI to an entire department or your whole company, along with the manual about interpreting the results correctly, go here: http://www.mindgarden. com/117-maslach-burnout-inventory.

Self-test. Four medical researchers boiled the MBI down to its essence, and tested their brief set of questions against the full MBI. They found that these two questions yielded pretty much the same results as giving the full MBI. If you agree with either of the following statements, you likely have at least one dimension of burnout:

- I feel burned out from my work.
- I have become more callous toward people since I took this job.

In addition, there are online sources for other, non-research-tested burnout self-tests. To take a sample interactive self-test, go here: https:// www.mindtools.com/pages/article/newTCS_08.htm.

Your Personal Warning Signs

We wrote this book for two reasons, to help you recover from burnout and to help you stay recovered. Without understanding these two important parts, as we each discovered to our own personal distress, burnout can be cyclical: recovery happens because you get out of the situation that was causing it (for instance, you graduate from your professional school or program) and you get some significant rest and care. Then burnout sneaks up on you again some years later.

As we dug through the medical research and built our system described in this book, we began to be very intentional about walking our talk, so that we wouldn't fall back into burnout again. After all, since life continually presents challenges and difficulties, were we remembering to apply our new skills?

The first step, we realized, was to recognize the signs. We wondered how we could notice we were beginning to lose it (just a little) under stress. For Beth, major signs included spraining her right ankle yet *again*, as well as many less-traumatic falls and scrapes. Once Beth had her burnout more under control, she was able to identify personal warning signs that occurred earlier in the process: snapping at her children and husband, resentfully wanting extra-special coddling and concentration becoming difficult. Marnie's warning signs included swearing in traffic, getting sick more frequently, and crying (for no apparent reason) on her way to work.

Here is a useful list of categories of behavioral warning signs from the Harvard HelpGuide about burnout (used with permission):

- Withdrawing from responsibilities

- Isolating yourself from others

- Procrastinating, taking longer to get things done

- Using food, drugs, or alcohol to cope

- Taking out your frustrations on others

- Skipping work or coming in late and leaving early

Interactive: What Are Your Warning Signs?

As you read about warning signs, what personal behavioral indicators have you become aware of, which warn you that you've been dealing with too much stress for too long? List them here. You'll come back to them later (in Chapter 11.)

Why Does My Burnout Seem Different?

Do you feel that your burnout is not quite fitting into the descriptions you've read so far?

This is a common feeling. One big reason: some researchers have concluded that the definition of burnout includes three distinct *types* of burnout, each with a distinctive root cause. If you read one of these descriptions and say, "Hey, that's me!" then hopefully the extra information about the root cause will help guide your recovery to your specific needs.

We both can testify from our personal experiences that these types of burnout feel rather different from each other.

Three Types of Burnout

Burnout Type Description	Recovery Goal
Frenetic Working increasingly harder and harder, despite being exhausted, in a desperate attempt to find success or a sense of satisfaction that can balance out the stress caused by the efforts you have already invested. This type tends to have a very inflexible approach to success.	*Change personal definition of success. Skills from the Burnout Shield system also helpful.*
Worn-out Exhaustion, pessimism and a sense of "why bother?" This usually results from a situation featuring difficult problems that don't usually have positive outcomes. It's especially common when the supervising authorities have a narrow definition of success, and fail to recognize effort and dedication.	*Build skills from the Burnout Shield system.*

Underchallenged	
A detached, unmotivated, indifferent work attitude. This can result from a monotonous or unstimulating work environment. Or, it can result from being worn down by the cumulative effects of dealing with a situation that feels beyond personal control.	*Major recovery goal: Find or create better match for your skills, interests and values. Skills from the Burnout Shield system also helpful.*

TABLE 3.2 The three subtypes of burnout; first described by psychologist Barry A. Farber

Let's take a quick look at all three types.

Frenetic Burnout

In frenetic burnout, the strongest feeling is that of not being able to make a difference. The person feeling this type of burnout tends to respond by increasing their efforts, doing still more, and more and more.

Worn-out Burnout

Worn-out burnout is "classic" burnout, the kind where you've lost your drive, your productivity, and your energy. It is the most profound burnout, and takes the most variety of skills to climb out of it and stay out.

Underchallenged Burnout

Underchallenged burnout comes from the long-term effects of not seeing any path forward in your personal or professional development. This is also sometimes referred to as "boreout" as in, "burned out from being chronically bored."

	Frenetic	**Worn-Out**	**Underchallenged**
Dedication to Work	Ambitious, Workaholic	Intermediate	Indifferent
Effort Level	Overload	Exhausted	Going through the motions
Locus of Control	External or Internal	External	External
Acknowledg-ment	May be present	Missing	Missing
Hope for the Future	High	Gone	Not an option
Dominant Feeling	I can get that good feeling back if I just do more!	Pessimism	Boredom
Brain Fog	Possible	May be severe	Possible
Hours Worked	Long	Long	May be long
Work Type	Demanding	Challenging, little control over results; or basic rules change unpredictably	Monotonous, glass ceiling, or temporary assignment
Increased Risk	1–3 years in job	3–10+ years in job	3 years or less in job

TABLE 3.3 Characteristics of the three burnout types

Note: "Locus of control" refers to the extent to which you feel in control of the events that shape your life. Having an external locus of control means you feel you do not have control.

Beth: My Frenetic Burnout Story

I had frenetic burnout during my first year in nursing grad school, a 3-year specialty program for non-nurse college graduates. The important part, for my frenetic burnout story? The part about learning as much as I could of RN nursing in eleven fast-paced months; a program that normally lasts 4 years.

As I completed each 8–10 week rotation that year, my respect for nurses grew exponentially. But it was also clear to me that as a "green" student nurse, I certainly could not make much of a difference to my patients in any of those clinical experiences. (Though I surely tried.) By the summer rotations, I felt like one of the walking wounded.

Recovery, for me, simply involved being done with that marathon year, resting through the one-month break allowed, and being allowed to begin studying for my beloved specialty. As a result, I didn't learn a thing that would help me be more resilient when burnout surfaced in my life again. I had toughed it out and survived. That's all I knew. And all I thought I needed to know.

Beth: My Worn-out Burnout Story

For me, this kind of burnout started about year 10 of my nurse-midwifery career. My worn-out burnout deepened, in troughs and waves, until I finally quit the field, about a decade later. Along the way, I spent a year on full medical disability.

Throughout this time, the only response I knew to my deepening exhaustion was pushing myself harder. I was baffled as the pushing became less and less effective. (As a nurse-midwife, had I seen the implications of my own metaphor at the time, I might have learned something important. In labor, successful pushing has a rhythm: push hard, rest deeply, push hard, rest deeply. In fact, as a midwife I could have carried the metaphor even further and learned even more. Midwives know that *gentle* pushing, in some situations, is as effective, and far safer, than pushing hard. But, sadly for me, I didn't make those connections until long after I left the field.)

Beth: My Underchallenged Burnout Story

I went through a couple of years of "boreout" when I was struggling vainly to make a success of a franchise I had purchased.

I felt that it was a wonderful company selling truly excellent products; I was proud to represent them. In the process of building my business, I learned a great deal both about nutrition and about business. Yet in truth, my skills and interests and the franchise's business system were only a very partial match.

Eventually, I hit a performance plateau; the more I struggled, the more I stayed stuck. I flailed and flailed, all the while sinking into a morass of brain fog and poor productivity, while wondering—once again—what was wrong with me. When I learned about Underchallenged burnout, I was incredibly relieved. I was so glad to have an explanation that fit my situation, but did not involve believing that I was somehow a bad person.

Very soon thereafter, I was able to walk away from that business, with all good will and gratitude, but also with a clear understanding that my *incomplete personal fit* with the franchise's business model had created my performance plateau, and the plateau in turn generated my boreout.

What Now?

As we have discussed earlier, each type of burnout can masquerade as other problems. You may have been chasing those other problems, not knowing they are all part of the bigger picture of burnout.

Now that you know the details about what burnout is and how it is affecting you, let's dive into what you can do about it.

Part II

Create Your Action Plan

Chapter FOUR

What Stands Between You and Burnout: Five Key Areas

Now that you understand more about burnout, what causes it and how to spot it, it is time to learn about how to protect yourself from it. In this chapter, we help you recognize the parts of your life that protect you from burnout. We call these areas the Five Key Areas.

Marnie: Our Discovery of the Five Key Areas

When you first decide to do something about your own burnout, it can be hard to know where to start. I remember the very moment when I decided to push past my own sense of helplessness to find a path that would make sense. I had been lecturing in front of a classroom of 112 medical students, discussing the topic of professional burnout. Using a self-test based on a modified Maslach Burnout Inventory, we had all just calculated our burnout risk scores.

I noticed that the room had grown very quiet. I looked out at them, and said, my own voice a bit shaky, "So, please raise your hand only if you feel comfortable sharing your score; how many of you are in the low risk category?" Nobody raised their hands.

"Moderate risk?" A couple people raised their hands.

"High risk?" A dozen or so raised their hands.

"Extremely high risk?" The entire rest of the room slowly raised their hands, as did I.

I saw tears well up in many students' eyes. There seemed to be a shared sense of vulnerability, compassion and relief, as well as fear. It was a powerful moment; for the first time, many of us were admitting to ourselves as well as to each other that our smooth exteriors were covering up a lot of pain inside.

I said, "Wow, this is serious, isn't it?"

One woman called out from the corner of the lecture hall, "But Dr. Loomis, what do we *do* about it?"

I realized that everything I had prepared for the lecture that day was focused on organizational causes of burnout. None of it was about how individuals could recover from burnout.

From that point forward, I started compiling the information and presenting workshops to various audiences. It became evident that many people were suffering from burnout or were dangerously close to it, and they were desperate for information about how they could get better.

When I met Beth Genly, I was thrilled to find another person who shared my passion for the topic. We decided to work together to develop a comprehensive recovery system for people who were suffering from burnout.

We agreed to keep in mind that people with burnout are exhausted and have little or no energy to spare. We realized we needed to develop a comprehensive, individualized system, not just tips and tricks. Otherwise, it could be difficult to prioritize what to do first, second, etc.

As a person with burnout, if I was going to do something to help myself, I wanted to know where it was most crucial to start, what the expected results would be, what I should be planning next. I would need to know that I wasn't somehow going to be making my problem worse by spending energy on something that wouldn't matter in the short term. I also didn't want to make the problem worse by exhausting myself more.

We also agreed that we needed to help people identify what aspects of their lives were protecting them, so they could justify continuing to do what they were already doing well. Otherwise, it would be too easy for someone to unintentionally cut something out of their lives that was actually protecting them. For instance, a person might hear the tip, "Improve time management to reduce stress and burnout." As a result, that person may cut out their lunch break in order to get more work done. But in the big picture of burnout, this move could be harmful in several ways, by affecting their overall nutrition, their social interaction time with colleagues and by interrupting a chance for mid-day physical activity.

We looked at hundreds of studies on stress and burnout and focused on ones that looked at populations where some people burned out and others didn't. What were the differences between these groups of people? Specifically, we were looking for studies that looked at things within the individual's control. Why did some people burn out while others did not, even though they were in the same situations? As we compiled the data from these studies, we found there were five Key Areas of a person's life that protected them from burnout: **their practice of self-care, their habits of reflection and recognition, their awareness of how close they are to their own maximum functional capacity, their involvement in their community, and their primary methods of coping.**

Overview of the Five Key Areas

The **Self-Care Key Area** looks at whether you are taking care of yourself and the basic functions that keep your body going. This includes eating, sleeping, hydration, elimination, sleep — all of the basic functions, which if you skip them now and then, aren't a big deal; but become a big deal if they are regularly interrupted or ignored.

Not everyone is good at knowing when they've given up too much. Nobody is surprised when a car that is out of gas stops running, but somehow many people expect their bodies to keep functioning even when they skip multiple meals, etc. If you haven't taken care of yourself, you aren't going to be much good to anyone else. Your own needs are a justifiable priority.

The Self-Care Key Area also includes whether you are doing your regular health maintenance. This includes seeing a doctor, dentist, psychologist or any other type of healthcare professional who is trained to address and treat any health problems you may have. The bottom line is that there are a lot of very common physical and mental health conditions that can reduce your capacity to deal with any type of stress. If you get them treated, then they don't have to be a limitation, but if these conditions are undiagnosed, or diagnosed but not well managed, they can severely impact your ability to deal with stress and avoid burnout.

Lastly, this Self-Care Key Area also includes some of the attitudes you may have about yourself, specifically, attitudes that might lead you to ignore or downplay the importance of your own needs. By pointing these attitudes out, the intention is not to assign blame, but rather to highlight the need for you to justify placing a high priority on your own needs.

The **Reflection and Recognition Key Area** includes some of the most powerful burnout-protective elements. Thankfully, this section also includes some of the least labor-intensive elements as well. Yes, you read that right! Some of the most positive things you can do to save yourself from burnout require very little energy to do.

As we discussed in Chapter 2, your brain is wired to use either your Reflective or your Reactive network to deal with all the information you have coming at you on a moment-by-moment basis. When your brain uses the Reflective network as your default network, you have many burnout-protective advantages. With your Reflective network in charge, you have greater overall endurance, the pain you experience is less intense and lasts for shorter periods of time, and you have an increased ability to reason, control your emotional responses and think of creative solutions to problems.

So the big question is: how do you put your Reflective network in charge? The neurology concept of "You wire what you fire," tells us that, depending on which network you use most often, your body will reinforce that network as the default network. Yes, you physically make changes to yourself to strengthen the connections you are using most often.

If you are currently burned out or are close to burning out, your Reactive network is most likely set as your default network. However, it is possible to override this default setting by *choosing* to use the Reflective network of your brain. By adopting regular reflective practices and training your mind over time, you can eventually reset your brain to put your Reflective network back in charge. The questions in the Reflection and Recognition Key Area look at the frequency with which you are using your Reflective or Reactive brain networks.

They also look at your level of awareness of your own feelings and values, whether the people around you recognize your accomplishments, and whether you allow yourself to observe things for what they are, even if you don't understand them.

In the **Capacity Key Area**, we look at elements indicating how much stress you can take on and your awareness of how close you are to that limit. In other words, have you spread yourself too thin? If you are spread too thin, are you aware of it? Another aspect we consider here is whether or not you are in a high-risk environment for burnout.

The Capacity Key Area is a little different than the other four, because a lot of what we are measuring isn't necessarily within your control.

However, what is in within your control is your *awareness* of your own capacity.

People tend to struggle in this area for many reasons. They may simply be stoic and ignore their own signs of distress with a "Put your head down and power through," attitude. Or they may think of their own energy in different silos, and not realize that the energy they expend at work and the energy they expend at home are both coming out of the same source.

Sometimes people also have a tendency to have a "no pain, no gain," attitude, and think that success will only come at the cost of personal comfort. While there can be something said for the value of setting high standards and working hard to achieve them, it is also important to recognize that this is not the same as setting totally unreasonable expectations of yourself.

Consider this analogy: let's say you have a delivery service. You've got a vehicle and you get offered all sorts of delivery jobs. Which jobs do you take on? That really depends on your capacity to take on cargo, which depends on a lot of other considerations. First of all, what kind of vehicle do you have? Is it a bike, a car, or a pickup truck? Was there previous damage to your vehicle that impacts how much it can carry? Are there outside considerations? Are you traveling on land or by water? What are the conditions of the roads? Are there tolls and fees that might limit how much you can take down the road? In order to take on new jobs, you'll need to have a good idea of your vehicle's capacity so that you can reach your destination with you and your cargo in one piece. Similarly, in life, it is good to be aware of your own functional Capacity so that you have a decent chance of successfully completing your tasks.

This section looks at some of the many elements of life that may impact your ability to take on additional stress. In medical science, the study of "allostatic load," looks at the physical wear and tear on a person's body that comes with repeated exposure to different kinds of stress. We take into consideration stressful life events as well as other elements that studies have shown might impact a person's allostatic load.

Of course, every person is different. Aspects such as resiliency, coping skills and a strong community may impact how much of a lasting effect a particular stressful event might actually have on you. Evaluating these elements for yourself will give you a better idea of your overall functional capacity.

If you have maxed out your Capacity, or are in an especially high-risk environment for burnout, it is time to start increasing your protective aspects in the remaining four areas as you work on the aspects that are within your control.

In the **Community Key Area**, we look at social elements in your life. Do you feel connected with a community of people who share your values and have good intentions for your well-being? If you do, are you having enough interaction with them? As you complete the Burnout Shield Self-Tests in Chapter 5, you will notice that we look at several different possible types of relationships. We also look at whether the natures of these relationships and the types of interactions you have within them are ones that are likely to help to protect you from burnout or whether they potentially increase your vulnerability.

Lastly, the **Coping Skills Key Area** looks at which types of coping methods you tend to use and whether they are actually helping you, or instead adding to the overall problem. This includes elements of how you actively deal with stress, as well as possible unconscious habits that you may not have realized were also types of coping methods.

When it comes to coping skills, there isn't a way to say absolutely that any one method is good or bad, as it really depends on the situation. However, depending on your type of burnout, there are some coping methods that are much more likely to add to your overall problem and others that are far more likely to actually bring relief and lower your overall stress burden. We discuss strategies for how to choose in Chapter 10.

As we read deeper and deeper into the burnout research literature, Beth and I realized why a simple list of "tips and tricks" never seemed to be enough when it came to dealing with burnout. People and situations vary greatly. We needed to develop a comprehensive yet individualized way for people to visualize what was most important to consider in their road to burnout recovery.

Introducing the Burnout Shield

We eventually created the Burnout Shield Self-Tests and the Burnout Shield, a visual "dashboard" of sorts that allowed people to do a quick visual assessment of their strongest and most vulnerable five Key Areas. It highlights *specific* areas of a person's life to improve or protect.

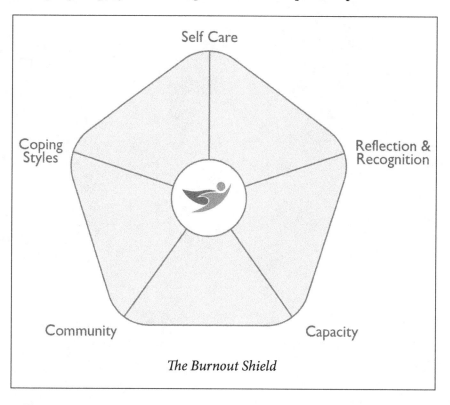

The Burnout Shield

In the next chapter, you will assess your own personal Burnout Shield. Be sure to do that assessment before moving on in the book. Doing the Self-Tests in Chapter 5 will tell you exactly where you need to start in Chapters 6–10, which discuss strategies for addressing each of your five Key Areas.

Chapter FIVE

Where Are You Strong? Where Are You Vulnerable? Your Burnout Shield Self-Tests

Now it is time to get everything out in the open! These five Burnout Shield Key Area Self-Tests will lead you through the process of examining which parts of your life may be protecting you and which may be leaving you the most vulnerable to burnout. Once you've established your Key Area scores, you can use them to help gain perspective on where to focus your efforts as you move forward to save yourself from burnout.

Please keep in mind that this is an informal tool intended only as a guide. We urge you to use common sense as you interpret the results. Consider any influential area of your life that may be underrepresented by this test and adjust your results accordingly. The Burnout Shield Self-Tests do not comprise a "validated" tool: they are not intended for diagnostic purposes, as they have not been put through rigorous, controlled scientific tests.

To our knowledge, no more rigorous, validated tests of this type yet exist, which is why we wrote this book in the first place. We hope you find them helpful in your quest for health and would appreciate your feedback, so we can improve them for future editions.

First, you'll fill out the five Key Area Self-Tests of the Burnout Shield, to come up with your starting scores in each Key Area. Then you'll learn how to easy it is to convert your own data to a visual map. **We call this map your Burnout Shield, because it shows at a glance in which areas you've built effective barriers against burnout, and where you have yet to do so**. Here's a sample Burnout Shield sketch, showing someone's five Key Areas. Your Burnout Shield is likely to have a far different shape, though, because you will have customized yours to your situation.

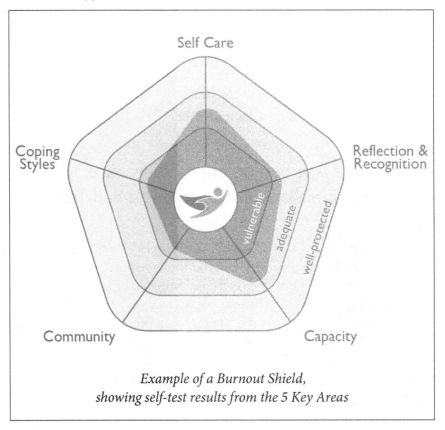

Example of a Burnout Shield,
showing self-test results from the 5 Key Areas

In the future, when your skills or circumstances change, we encourage you to come back to this chapter and do a new set of Key Area Self-Tests for yourself. This is a great way to **track your progress, re-commit to skills that might have slipped, and celebrate your accomplishments**.

Please **allow yourself to be super-candid** when you're answering the five Key Area Self-Tests. No-one will see your answers unless you choose to share them, and of course you'll get the most out of these assessments when you are honest with yourself.

Also, please, **be gentle with yourself.** While answering these questions, you may discover you've been making choices that contribute to the development of your own burnout or that harmed you in some other way. Please remember to acknowledge that harsh judgment will only cause more harm. Make yourself this promi: *gentle with myself during this process.*

REMEMBER: *Please do not consider these as value judgments or contests. You are gathering information about where you are right now.*

The Self-Care Key Area

Value Yourself
How high a priority do you set on your own health and wellbeing? As you learned in Part I, stress has major effects on your body, and burnout severely impacts your productivity, your energy, and even your ability to enjoy life. Here is where you get to identify some specifics. Ask yourself:

Am I treating myself as if I were a robot or a machine? Or am I remembering to regularly rejuvenate my human energy?

Self-Care Self-Test

Instructions
Write the letter of the multiple choice answer that most represents your present situation. Write that letter (A, B, C, or D) on the line to the right of its question. At the end, you'll get instructions on how to score this Key Area. Toward the end of this chapter, you'll also map each of your Key Area scores onto your Burnout Shield.

My sleep...
A. My sleep is erratic, brief, and often interrupted.
B. I occasionally sleep well, but I generally sleep 6 hours a night or less.
C. I sleep well some nights every week. I generally sleep 7–8 hours at night.
D. I sleep well most nights every week. I generally sleep 7–8 hours at night.

_____

I eat regular meals...

A. I frequently skip meals or eat snack food instead of meals.
B. Sporadically; I sometimes delay or skip meals.
C. Some days of the week.
D. Most days of the week. _____

The kind of food I eat is...

A. Mostly fast food, snack food or vending machine food.
B. Whatever is convenient, occasionally healthy.
C. Sometimes healthy, sometimes just convenient.
D. Mostly healthy. _____

My exercise habits are...

A. I am nearly completely sedentary.
B. Several times a day, I get up and move around a bit more than just shifting from chair to chair.
C. A few times a week, I exercise for at least 20–30 minutes.
D. In some way, nearly every day, I exercise for at least 20–30 minutes. _____

Regarding my physical and mental health issues...

A. I've not seen a health care professional within the last year, and my health issues are moderately or severely troublesome.
B. I've not seen a health care professional within the last year, and my health issues are mildly or moderately troublesome.
C. I'm actively working with my health care professional this year to get my health issues under control.
D. I have seen a health care professional this year; I don't have any health issues or my health issues are well managed. _____

I spend time with family and friends...

A. On major holidays.
B. A few times a month.
C. At least once a week.
D. Several times a week. _____

(Self-Care Self-Test, continued)

Regarding the separation of work time and personal time...

    A. I'm on call 24/7; work issues frequently interrupt my personal time.

    B. Work issues often interrupt my personal time.

    C. I am sometimes able to have uninterrupted personal time.

    D. I am frequently able to have uninterrupted personal time. _____

Regarding my ability to take care of my personal needs, such as bathroom breaks...

    A. I'm so used to ignoring my own needs that I barely notice them anymore.

    B. I often have to delay my personal needs because I'm too busy.

    C. I sometimes have to delay my personal needs because I'm too busy.

    D. I'm able to stop and take care of my needs as they occur. _____

Regarding my sense of compassion for myself (and how I handle my challenges or failures)...

    A. I don't have much compassion for myself and often get down on myself for my failures.

    B. I hadn't really considered whether I have compassion for myself.

    C. I have a moderate amount of compassion for myself.

    D. I have a strong sense of compassion for myself. _____

Regarding judgment about myself and my feelings...

    A. I am much harder on myself than anyone else is; I frequently use self-talk that is sarcastic and negative.

    B. I sometimes find myself using self-talk that is sarcastic and negative.

    C. I sometimes tell myself I should be happy and shouldn't be feeling these negative feelings.

    D. I am frequently non-judgmental about my feelings, whatever they may be. _____

Calculate your total Self-Care score:

A= 1 point, B= 2 points, C= 3 points, D= 4 points.

Your Score:	Vulnerable	Adequate	Well-Protected
	10–20	21–30	31–40

If your Self-Care Key Area score falls in the range 10–20: To make burnout a thing of the past, Self-Care will be very fruitful for you to address. It's likely you've been pushing yourself unmercifully, and either ignoring your body's signals or simply not being conscious of them. Getting good at responding in a timely way to these signals, so that you engage in renewal *before* you wear out, is like building a new muscle group: it takes time, patience, commitment and most of all, the ability to go easy on yourself. **Protection: Vulnerable**

If your Self-Care Key Area score falls in the range 21–30: You've got some good Self-Care skills (more about them in Chapter 6). Adding some more skills to your repertoire would likely be of value, but if some of your other Key Areas are at a Vulnerable level, you needn't make this Area your first focus in your shift toward a burnout-free lifestyle. Just be aware the Self-Care skills you're already using are highly valuable. Remember to do a quick mental review of this Self-Care Key Area of your Burnout Shield when high-pressure situations arise, to make sure you're not inadvertently under-prioritizing those skills you're already good at. **Protection: Adequate**

If your Self-Care Key Area score falls in the range 31–40: Congratulations, you are doing a great job! Again, when high-pressure situations arise, remember to quickly review your activities in this key area of your Burnout Shield to make sure you're not inadvertently giving short shrift to these Self-Care key area skills which you're already so good at. **Protection: Well-Protected**

The Reflection & Recognition Key Area

Reflect Daily; Recognize Even Small Accomplishments
How frequently do you reflect on your accomplishments and what is meaningful to you? The Reflection and Recognition Key Area of your

Burnout Shield assesses your awareness of your feelings and those around you; your sense of meaning and purpose, and the amount and style of recognition you receive — and give yourself — for your good work.

This Key Area of the Shield can be a low effort/high payoff realm in which to make changes. Research shows that shifting the focus of your attention for even a few minutes each day to reflect on meaning and personal values actually shifts your brain into more functional pathways, while soothing your stressed body systems. In brief, ask yourself:

How can I honor my own values today?

Reflection & Recognition Self-Test

Instructions

Write the letter of the multiple choice answer that most represents your present situation. Write that letter (A, B, C, or D) on the line to the right of its question. At the end, you'll get instructions on how to score this Key Area. Toward the end of this chapter, you'll also map each of your Key Area scores onto your Burnout Shield.

Regarding my level of engagement in my work...
   A. I don't like my work, or I feel disillusioned about it.
   B. I feel indifferent about my work.
   C. I feel somewhat engaged in my work.
   D. I feel very engaged in my work.   _____

I reflect back on the meaningful events that happened during the day...
   A. Rarely or never.
   B. Occasionally.
   C. Sometimes.
   D. Frequently.   _____

Regarding life and its meaning...
   A. I feel like my life is meaningless.
   B. I'm indifferent about whether or not my life has meaning.
   C. I have a good sense that my life has meaning.
   D. I have a clear sense that my life has meaning.   _____

At work, most often the type of recognition I receive is the type I prefer and enjoy. (Examples: public recognition, private/verbal acknowledgement, awards, or token gifts)...
A. Rarely or never (*or,* I do not receive recognition.)
B. Occasionally.
C. Sometimes.
D. Frequently.   _____

My supervisor/coworkers stop to recognize my accomplishments or our shared accomplishments...
A. Rarely or never.
B. Occasionally.
C. Sometimes.
D. Frequently.   _____

I stop to recognize and acknowledge my own accomplishments...
A. Rarely or never.
B. Occasionally.
C. Sometimes.
D. Frequently.   _____

Regarding goal setting and definition of success (note: even if you don't currently set goals, please answer in the way that is most like you)...
A. I set extremely tough goals and have a very rigid definition of success.
B. I set fairly tough goals and have a somewhat rigid definition of success.
C. I set fairly achievable goals and have a somewhat flexible definition of success.
D. I set extremely achievable goals and have a very flexible definition of success.   _____

Regarding my level of awareness of my own feelings (happiness, sadness, etc.) and sensations (heart racing, muscle tension, etc.)...
   A. I feel numb or disconnected from my own feelings and sensations.
   B. I am rarely aware of my own feelings and sensations.
   C. I am sometimes aware of my own feelings and sensations.
   D. I am frequently aware of my own feelings and sensations. _____

Regarding how I deal with my own feelings...
   A. I usually try to avoid unpleasant feelings and am extremely self-critical.
   B. I occasionally try to avoid unpleasant feelings and am rather self-critical.
   C. I am somewhat accepting of all my feelings and only occasionally self-critical.
   D. I am fully accepting of all my feelings and rarely self-critical. _____

Regarding my awareness of my own injuries...
   A. I frequently get hurt and don't even notice it until much later.
   B. If I injure myself, I am sometimes aware of it.
   C. If I injure myself, I am usually aware of it.
   D. If I injure myself, I am immediately aware of it. _____

Regarding a spiritual, religious, or daily meditation practice...
   A. I don't have any spiritual, religious or daily meditation practice or beliefs.
   B. I practice this sometimes.
   C. I practice this often.
   D. I practice this daily. _____

Calculate your total Reflection & Recognition score:

A= 1 point, B= 2 points, C= 3 points, D= 4 points.

Your Score:	Vulnerable	Adequate	Well-Protected
	11–22	23–34	35–44

If your Reflection & Recognition Key Area score falls in the range of 11–22: Tune in! Just adding a few minutes of reflection and attention to feelings each day may give you a powerful boost. Building some good Recognition and Reflection skills principally requires a shift in mindset. **Protection: Vulnerable**

If your Reflection & Recognition Key Area score falls in the range of 23–34: Pat yourself on the back! You've got some good Reflection & Recognition skills. Adding some more Reflection & Recognition skills to your repertoire would likely be of value in your shift into a burnout-free lifestyle, but if other areas are more vulnerable you don't need to make the Reflection and Recognition key area your first focus. Just be aware that the skills which you're already using are highly valuable. When high-pressure situations arise, do a quick mental review of this area of your Burnout Shield, to make sure you're not inadvertently under-utilizing Reflection & Recognition key area skills in times of crisis. **Protection: Adequate**

If your Reflection & Recognition Key Area score falls in the range of 35–44: High five! Congratulations, you rock at Reflection & Recognition skills. Again, when high-pressure situations arise, remember to quickly review your activities in this Key Area of your Burnout Shield to make sure you're not suddenly underusing your simple but powerful Reflection & Recognition skills. **Protection: Well-Protected**

The Capacity Key Area

Start Small

Given your situation and your internal characteristics (which are, for the most part, things that are out of your control) what is your vulnerability to burnout?

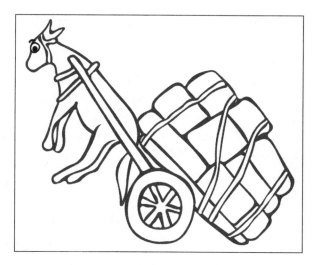

Look at this picture of what happens when this poor donkey tries to pull an overloaded cart. In the spirit of this picture, we like to think of your Capacity Key Area as the "donkey cart" you're pulling. **What's in your cart? Is it reasonable to expect yourself to pull that much?**

If you prefer a more modern analogy, visualize a car that's been so overloaded its doors can't be shut, the driver is about to lose control, the car itself may break down, and its riders are not safe. **Have you loaded yourself past your Capacity?**

You might also consider: did the person who chose to overload that car actually improve their situation when they decided not to rent to borrow a truck for the day? What kind of vehicle are you driving? **Can your "vehicle" carry the load you've heaped on it?**

To get a full picture of the load on your Capacity, you'll complete two Self-Tests:

- Holmes and Rahe Life Stress Inventory
- Capacity Key Area Self-Test

You'll do the Holmes and Rahe Life Stress Inventory first. By the way, this stress assessment, developed by two brilliant scientists named, not too surprisingly, Holmes and Rahe, has been shown repeatedly to predict one's risk for a "health breakdown" over the next two years (as you'll see at the bottom of the stress inventory.)

NOTE: The Holmes and Rahe Life Stress Inventory is by no means a *complete* list of major life stressors. You may well have experienced (or are still undergoing) an important life stressor that is not on this list.

The Holmes and Rahe Life Stress Inventory

Instructions

Circle the point value of each of these life events that has happened to you during the previous year. Total these associated points.

Once you've calculated your Holmes and Rahe Life Stress Inventory score, then you'll plug it into the appropriate question in the second part, the Capacity Key Area Self-Test.

	Life Event	Mean Value
1.	Death of spouse	100
2.	Divorce	73
3.	Marital separation from mate	65
4.	Detention in jail or other institution	63
5.	Death of a close family member	63
6.	Major personal injury or illness	53
7.	Marriage	50
8.	Being fired at work	47
9.	Marital reconciliation with mate	45
10.	Retirement from work	45
11.	Major change in the health or behavior of a family member	44
12.	Pregnancy	40
13.	Sexual difficulties	39
14.	Gaining a new family member (i.e., birth, adoption, older adult moving in, etc.)	39
15.	Major business readjustment	39
16.	Major change in financial state (i.e., a lot worse or better off than usual)	38
17.	Death of a close friend	37
18.	Changing to a different line of work	36
19.	Major change in the number of arguments with spouse (i.e., either a lot more or a lot less than usual regarding child rearing, personal habits, etc.)	35

20.	Taking on a mortgage (for home, business, etc.)	31
21.	Foreclosure on a mortgage or loan	30
22.	Major change in responsibilities at work (i.e., promotion, demotion, etc.)	29
23.	Son or daughter leaving home (i.e., marriage, attending college, joined mil.)	29
24.	In-law troubles	29
25.	Outstanding personal achievement	28
26.	Spouse beginning or ceasing work outside the home	26
27.	Beginning or ceasing formal schooling	26
28.	Major change in living condition (new home, remodeling, deterioration of neighborhood or home, etc.)	25
29.	Revision of personal habits (dress, manners, associations, quitting smoking)	24
30.	Troubles with the boss	23
31.	Major changes in working hours or conditions	20
32.	Changes in residence	20
33.	Changing to a new school	20
34.	Major change in usual type and/or amount of recreation	19
35.	Major change in church activity (i.e., a lot more or less than usual)	19
36.	Major change in social activities (clubs, movies, visiting, etc.)	18
37.	Taking on a loan (car, TV, freezer, etc.)	17
38.	Major change in sleeping habits (a lot more or a lot less than usual)	16
39.	Major change in number of family get-togethers	15
40.	Major change in eating habits (a lot more or less food intake, or very different meal hours or surroundings)	15
41.	Vacation	13
42.	Major holidays	12
43.	Minor violations of the law (traffic tickets, jaywalking, disturbing the peace, etc.)	11

Now, add up all the points you've circled to find your Holmes and Rahe score.
_____

150 points or less means a relatively low amount of life changes and a low susceptibility to stress-induced health breakdown.

150 to 300 points implies about a 50% chance of a major health breakdown in the next 2 years.

301 points or more raises the odds to about 80% of a health breakdown in the next 2 years, according to the Holmes and Rahe prediction model.

Capacity Key Area Self-Test

Instructions
Write the letter of the multiple choice answer that most represents your present situation. Write that letter (A, B, C, or D) on the line to the right of its question. At the end, you'll get instructions on how to score this Key Area. Toward the end of this chapter, you'll also map each of your Key Area scores onto your Burnout Shield.

Today, my Holmes and Rahe Life Stress Inventory score fell in this range...
A. 300 or more.
B. 150–299.
C. 50–149.
D. 0–50.
_____

The typical stress level at my job or in my line of work (or educational program) is...
A. High.
B. Moderate.
C. Low.
D. Very low.
_____

(Capacity Key Area Self-Test, continued)

I participate in shift work (am assigned other than 9–5 hours)...
A. Frequently.
B. Sometimes.
C. Occasionally.
D. Infrequently or never.   _____

I'm formally on-call after hours...
A. Frequently.
B. Sometimes.
C. Occasionally.
D. Infrequently or never.   _____

I'm expected to respond to correspondence after hours...
A. Frequently.
B. Sometimes.
C. Occasionally.
D. Infrequently or never.   _____

I have a high level of responsibility to others outside of my work life (may include parenthood, primary caretaker responsibilities, community involvement, etc.)...
A. Frequently.
B. Sometimes.
C. Occasionally.
D. Infrequently or never.   _____

I have more than one job (or attend night school)...
A. Frequently.
B. Sometimes.
C. Occasionally.
D. Infrequently or never.   _____

(Capacity Key Area Self-Test, continued)

My typical work week (total) is...
    A. I work more than 50 hours a week.
    B. I work more 40–50 hours a week.
    C. I work about 40 hours a week.
    D. I work less than 35 hours a week.   _____

At work (or school), I clearly understand what is expected of me...
    A. Infrequently or never.
    B. Occasionally.
    C. Sometimes.
    D. Frequently.   _____

The workload expected of me seems reasonable...
    A. Infrequently or never.
    B. Occasionally.
    C. Sometimes.
    D. Frequently.   _____

I have enough resources (people, training, money, materials) to get the job done...
    A. Infrequently or never.
    B. Occasionally.
    C. Sometimes.
    D. Frequently.   _____

My job security is...
    A. Extremely poor: I am at risk of losing my job.
    B. Poor: I am somewhat at risk of losing my job.
    C. Good: Somewhat secure.
    D. Excellent: Highly secure.   _____

My pay level/reward in relation to my work is...
    A. Not enough.
    B. Somewhat low.
    C. Good.
    D. Very good.   _____

My autonomy level (level of control) at work is...

A. Extremely low.
B. Low.
C. Moderate.
D. High.　　　　　　　　　　　　　　　　_____

The sense of fairness at work (or school) is...

A. Extremely unfair.
B. Unfair.
C. Somewhat fair.
D. Very fair.　　　　　　　　　　　　　　　_____

The values where I work reflect my own values...

A. Infrequently or never.
B. Occasionally.
C. Sometimes.
D. Frequently.　　　　　　　　　　　　　　_____

The stress level related to my commute to and from work is...

A. High.
B. Moderate.
C. Low.
D. Extremely low.　　　　　　　　　　　　_____

Regarding my exposure to nature or images of nature during my work week...

A. No plants or nature scenes are visible near my work station or my home.
B. Pictured nature scenes are visible where I work.
C. I see healthy potted plants when I look up from my work.
D. I walk for at least 20 minutes through a park, large garden, or forested area several times a week.　　_____

(Capacity Key Area Self-Test, continued)

My financial stability is...
A. Very unstable.
B. Somewhat unstable.
C. Somewhat secure.
D. Highly secure.   ———

Regarding introversion (most comfortable alone) vs extroversion (most comfortable in groups)...
A. I'm extremely introverted.
B. I'm somewhat introverted.
C. I'm somewhat extroverted.
D. I'm extremely extroverted.   ———

Calculate your total Capacity score:

A= 1 point, B= 2 points, C= 3 points, D= 4 points.

Your Score:	Vulnerable	Adequate	Well-Protected
	20–40	41–60	61–80

If your Capacity Key Area score falls in the range of 20–40: **Lighten your load!** What can you drop from your load, even temporarily? If your cart is so overloaded that the donkey's feet can't touch the path; if your car is so full you can't shut the doors to drive, then something has to give. In order to make sure that what "gives" isn't your resilience and your health, it is really important that you lighten your load. **Protection: Vulnerable**

If your Capacity Key Area score falls in the range of 41–60: **Redistribute the load.** It may not be necessary to make this Area your first focus in your shift into a burnout-free lifestyle, if your scores show you are more vulnerable in other Areas. You might be doing okay for now, carrying the load you've got, but you still may need to adjust your priorities. What can you downgrade in priority or at least shift to a different time or day? Also, take note of the highly valuable Capacity skills that you are already using. Do a quick mental review of the Capacity Key Area of your Burnout Shield when high-pressure situations arise; especially make sure you're avoiding piling on to your load without also making room. **Protection: Adequate**

If your Capacity Key Area score falls in the range of 61–80: You're balanced! Your Capacity situation has a good chance of matching your ability to carry the load; possibly just minor tweaks are needed. As always, when your load becomes overwhelming or unstable, remember to quickly review your situation to see what you might delay, delegate or drop. **Protection: Well-Protected**

The Community Key Area

Ask for Help, Get Perspective
Do the people around you, and the nature of your relationships to them, help protect you, or make you more vulnerable to burnout?

Withdrawal from our connections with others, due to exhaustion or cynicism, or both, is part of the very definition of burnout. We usually withdraw to get relief from our emotional exhaustion. Sometimes our withdrawal from human contact is also fueled by an element of burnout-related guilt or grief. In other words, we withdraw to protect ourselves.

Unfortunately, that withdrawal further drives the vicious circle of burnout. Establishing or rebuilding your Community can take time and energy. This is why we place this Key Area fourth on the Burnout Shield: once you are renewing your energy and attention by upgrading your Self-Care, Reflection & Recognition, and Capacity skills, then Community skills may come a lot easier to you.

Your personality structure may also affect how easy it is for you to address the Community Key Area. Extroverts may like to start by tackling this. On the other hand, if you tend to be more introverted, you may not wish to start here in this Burnout Shield key area.

In brief, to do a quick assessment of this area, ask yourself:

Do the ways I interact create positive results for me and my community?

Community Key Area Self-Test

Instructions

Write the letter of the multiple choice answer that most represents your present situation. Write that letter (A, B, C, or D) on the line to the right of its question. At the end, you'll get instructions on how to score this Key Area. Toward the end of this chapter, you'll also map each of your Key Area scores onto your Burnout Shield.

Regarding my sense of connection with a supportive community...

A. I don't feel welcome in my community, or I feel targeted by others.

B. I'm not very connected to my community, but I feel like I'd be welcomed if I wanted to be.

C. I feel somewhat connected to my community.

D. I feel very connected to my community. _____

The sense of teamwork where I work is...

A. Non-existent: it is a cutthroat environment.

B. Doesn't apply.

C. Moderate.

D. Strong. _____

My relationship with my supervisor...

A. My supervisor doesn't seem to care if I work myself to the point of injury, or I have an outright conflict with my supervisor.

B. My supervisor seems to care only about my work, not its impact on my wellbeing.

C. My supervisor is somewhat supportive of my work and my overall wellbeing.

D. My supervisor is very supportive of my work and my overall well-being. _____

The level of respect I feel I get from those around me is...

A. Low; I don't feel respected by the people around me.

B. Mixed; I'm respected by some but not by others.

C. Good in general, but there are a few who are disrespectful.

D. In general, very high. _____

My closest personal relationship (family, spouse, partner, close friend) is...
A. Full of conflict and a source of stress.
B. I don't really have any close personal relationships.
C. Somewhat supportive and loving.
D. Extremely supportive and loving. _____

Regarding who takes care of whom within my community...
A. I am always the caretaker for others, they never take care of me.
B. I am usually the caretaker for others, they sometimes they take care of me.
C. I am usually the receiver of care in my community, I sometimes take care of others.
D. We care for one another in a fairly equal amount. _____

My communication skills are...
A. Poor.
B. Okay.
C. Good.
D. Great. _____

When it comes to asking for help...
A. I make it a point not to ask others for help.
B. I don't like asking others for help, but I can do it if I have to.
C. I can sometimes ask others for help.
D. I'm easily able to ask others for help. _____

When it comes to delegating tasks to others...
A. I do pretty much everything myself; I don't trust anyone else to do things for me.
B. I often tend to complete tasks myself; it's easier than asking others to do the work.
C. Occasionally I choose to complete something myself, even if someone else is willing and available.
D. I'm skilled at delegating tasks to others as appropriate. _____

When it comes to conflict resolution, I feel my skills are...
- A. Poor; I often snap at others, or have emotional outbursts.
- B. Fair; I tend to find myself in one conflict after another, or else I usually try to avoid conflict altogether.
- C. Good; I can address some issues, but sometimes I find I only make things worse.
- D. Excellent; I can address issues in a non-emotional way, and help find mutually beneficial solutions. _____

When I'm dealing with a problem, I seek out perspective from other people whose opinion I respect...
- A. Rarely or never.
- B. Sometimes.
- C. Often.
- D. Frequently. _____

Regarding the communication within my work community, the ratio of positive to negative comments is...
- A. Mostly negative: more negative than positive comments.
- B. Neutral: the same amount of negative and positive comments.
- C. Mildly positive: about two positive comments for every negative one.
- D. Mostly positive: more than three positive comments for every negative one. _____

At work, my coworkers spend time venting their frustrations...
- A. Frequently.
- B. Often.
- C. Sometimes.
- D. Rarely. _____

Calculate your total Community score:

A= 1 point, B= 2 points, C= 3 points, D= 4 points.

Your Score:	Vulnerable	Adequate	Well-Protected
	13–26	27–40	41–52

If your Community Key Area score falls in the range of 13-26: **Reach out!** When you're ready to give your attention to rebuilding key relationships, start by looking for someone who can offer perspective, possibly from outside your immediate work environment. There's more specifics on how to do this in Chapter 9. If this Area is a particular challenge for you, we'd also strongly urge you to find some support from a professional counselor or coach. **Protection: Vulnerable**

If your Community Key Area score falls in the range of 27-40: **Shake hands!** You're maintaining at least a few key relationships in good shape. While increasing your connections might feel good, you don't need to make this Key Area your first focus in your shift into a burnout-free lifestyle. Just be aware how highly valuable the skills you're already using are. Do a quick mental review of this Area of your Burnout Shield when high-pressure situations arise, to make sure you're not shutting out others when things get tough. **Protection: Adequate**

If your Community Key Area score falls in the range of 41-52: **Party!** Your relationships are in good shape. Again, when high-pressure situations arise, remember to quickly review your activities in this Key Area of your Burnout Shield to make sure you're not disconnecting from people who are crucial to your sense of Community. **Protection: Well-Protected**

The Coping Styles Key Area

Rethink Your Reactions
Am I creating distractions or diversions, instead of bringing my best resources to the problem?

Of course, there isn't a concrete way to say whether someone's coping mechanisms are "good" or "bad." It all depends on the situation. Here we ask you to consider, in your current situation, whether your coping mechanisms are helpful to you in the long run. Are they protective, or are they just adding to the overall problem?

For instance, when you are disappointed or grieving, an *emotion-focused* coping style is appropriate. Until you have recognized and processed your feelings sufficiently, grief or severe disappointment will suck down your energy and ability to move forward.

On the other hand, when you are facing a challenge, even if it carries an emotional charge for you, your best coping styles approach may be to reframe or reconstruct your view of the issue so that you can take a *problem-solving* approach.

Both coping styles, emotion-focused and problem-solving, can be useful when applied to the right situations.

In brief, quickly assess your Coping Styles Key Area by asking yourself:

Am I framing this issue in a way that allows me to address it most directly?

Coping Styles Self-Test

Instructions

Write the letter of the multiple choice answer that most represents your present situation. Write that letter (A, B, C, or D) on the line to the right of its question. At the end, you'll get instructions on how to score this Key Area. Toward the end of this chapter, you'll also map each of your Key Area scores onto your Burnout Shield.

When faced with a new challenge or something that upsets me, I pause and think before I act...
  A. Infrequently or never.
  B. Rarely.
  C. Sometimes.
  D. Frequently.   _____

When I feel like my stamina is fading while I'm working on an important task...
  A. I keep working and push myself harder.
  B. I'll rarely take a brief break.
  C. I'll sometimes take a brief break.
  D. I'll usually take a brief break and try to come back to
     the problem with a clear mind.   _____

When it comes to multitasking...
  A. I'm always multitasking. You should see how many other things I'm doing right now.
  B. I usually multitask, it seems to come with the job and I don't know how to stop it.
  C. I sometimes multitask but I stick to one task at a time when I'm crunched for time.
  D. I rarely multitask. I usually get one thing done and then move on to the next task. _____

I feel that the good and bad things that happen in my life are due to...
  A. Factors that are mostly beyond my control.
  B. Factors that are somewhat beyond my control.
  C. Somewhat my own efforts and hard work.
  D. Mostly my own efforts and hard work. _____

I'm open-minded and flexible when it comes to doing things in a new way (for example, I try to see things from other perspectives, consider different ways to solve problems)...
  A. Infrequently or never.
  B. Rarely.
  C. Sometimes.
  D. Frequently. _____

I seek the advice or perspective of others when I am feeling overwhelmed...
  A. Rarely or never.
  B. Sometimes.
  C. Often.
  D. Usually. _____

I allow others to help me...
  A. Just about never; I am the one who helps everyone else.
  B. Rarely.
  C. Sometimes.
  D. Frequently. _____

I have a practice that helps me feel grounded or connected to something larger than myself (such as a spiritual or religious practice)...

   A. No.

   B. Yes, and I practice them occasionally.

   C. Yes, and I practice them sometimes.

   D. Yes, and I practice them frequently.   _____

I use humor (with myself and others)...

   A. Just about never.

   B. Rarely.

   C. Sometimes.

   D. Frequently.   _____

I try to see the bright side or silver lining of a tough situation...

   A. Infrequently or never.

   B. Rarely.

   C. Sometimes.

   D. Frequently.   _____

When I'm stressed, I take part in solitary activities that sooth or comfort me such as a personal hobby or activity (video games, crafts, etc.)...

   A. Frequently, and it takes up a great deal of my time.

   B. Often, and it takes up a moderate amount of my time.

   C. Sometimes, and it takes up a small amount of my time.

   D. Occasionally, but it doesn't take up much of my time.   _____

I use regular exercise to manage my stress levels...

   A. Infrequently or never.

   B. Rarely.

   C. Sometimes.

   D. Frequently.   _____

I vent my negative feelings (anger, frustrations) to others...
A. Daily.
B. Often.
C. Occasionally.
D. Infrequently.

_____

I drink alcohol, smoke or do drugs...
A. Daily.
B. Often.
C. Occasionally.
D. Infrequently.

_____

Calculate your total Coping Styles score:

A= 1 point, B= 2 points, C= 3 points, D= 4 points.

Your Score:	Vulnerable	Adequate	Well-Protected
	14–28	29–43	44–56

If your Coping Styles Key Area score falls in the range of 14–28: Rethink your reactions. Earplugs and umbrellas are both examples of protective things that aren't exactly interchangeable. Coping Skills can be the same way. They are useful, but only if they are being used for the right situation. If your Coping Styles Key Area score is in this range, it is probably time for a reassessment. If this makes your head spin, it may help to seek some outside help as you go through this process. Thankfully, any improvements you make in this area are likely to be extremely rewarding. **Protection: Vulnerable**

If your Coping Styles Key Area score falls in the range of 29–43: Widen your scope. Adding some additional coping techniques might add to your resilience, but you don't need to make this Area your first focus in your shift into a burnout-free lifestyle. Just be aware how highly valuable these skills you're already using are. Do a quick mental review of this Area of your Burnout Shield when high-pressure situations arise; especially make sure you're avoiding venting or multitasking. **Protection: Adequate**

If your **Coping Styles Key Area score falls in the range of 44–56: You're flexible!** You usually vary your Coping Styles to suit the situation. Again, when high-pressure situations arise, remember to quickly review your activities in the Coping Styles Key Area of your Burnout Shield to make sure you're not losing flexibility as things get rough. **Protection: Well-Protected**

Create Your Burnout Shield

Great! You've completed scoring yourself in each of the five Burnout Shield Key Areas. We're proud of you for determining your scores for all five Burnout Shield Key Area Self-Tests. Good job! We're pretty sure that took patience, honesty, and persistence. Many people find it is emotionally stressful as well. Now you know what you're doing well, and you know the Key Areas most likely to trip you up.

Now, in this part of the chapter, you get to map your scores onto your Burnout Shield, which gives you a very personal, instant view of where you are protected from burnout, and where you are vulnerable. In turn, your Burnout Shield map gives you a clearer idea of where to start making improvements to help save yourself from burnout.

You might visualize your own Burnout Shield as the kind of shield a knight of old would carry, protecting you from the "slings and arrows of outrageous fortune." Yet again, you might see it in your mind's eye as a powerful futuristic force field, keeping you safe even from "photon torpedoes" and "energy weapons."

However you choose to carry your Burnout Shield in your mind, your job now is to get an idea of your Burnout Shield's present strength and coverage.

For your convenience, copy your five Self-Test Key Area scores and circle your protection levels here:

Self-Care

Your Score:	Vulnerable	Adequate	Well-Protected
	10–20	21–30	31–40

Reflection & Recognition

Your Score:	Vulnerable	Adequate	Well-Protected
	11–22	23–34	35–44

Capacity

Your Score:	Vulnerable	Adequate	Well-Protected
	20–40	41–60	61–80

Community

Your Score:	Vulnerable	Adequate	Well-Protected
	13–26	27–40	41–52

Coping Skills

Your Score:	Vulnerable	Adequate	Well-Protected
	14–28	29–43	44–56

How to Use Your Scores to Create Your Burnout Shield Map

Creating an "at a glance" version of your current Burnout Shield status can help you keep track of everything in a quick, easy way. To help you do that, we've created a blank version of the Burnout Shield map where you can plot your scores and draw your current Shield.

In the next few pages, we'll give you a quick description of how to do that — it's easy! Then, you'll use the scores you just recorded on the previous page, as you map your own Burnout Shield on page 82.

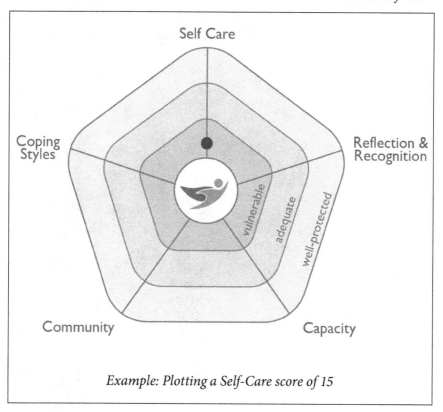

Example: Plotting a Self-Care score of 15

Step 1: Plot your scores on each axis. To start, put a dot on each axis of the Shield, corresponding to the protection level of each score. For example, if your Self-Care score is 15 (Vulnerable), then you'll place a dot in the Vulnerable zone, like this.

Once you've placed all five dots on the five Key Area axes, connect all five dots, and color in the shape you've just drawn.

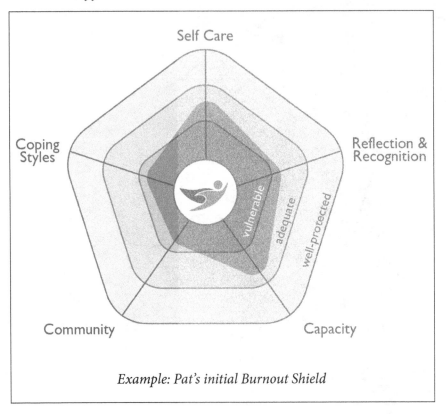

Example: Pat's initial Burnout Shield

Step 2: Connect the dots and color it in. For example, Pat's initial scores were Self Care: 25, Reflection and Recognition: 26, Capacity: 55, Community: 20, Coping: 25. Pat's initial Burnout Shield map looked like this.

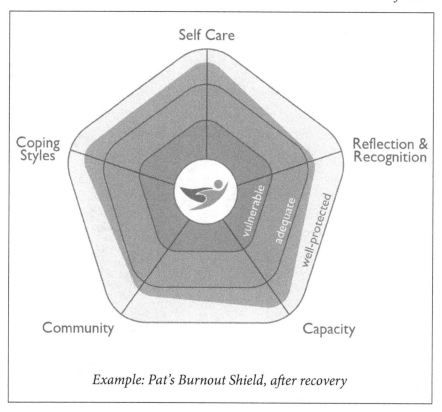

Example: Pat's Burnout Shield, after recovery

Step 3: Burnout Shield will change as you do. After several rounds of working through the rest of the chapters in this book and making gradual but strategic improvements, Pat's current scores are Self Care: 37, Reflection and Recognition: 38, Capacity: 72, Community: 44, Coping: 43. Pat's Burnout Shield map now looks like this.

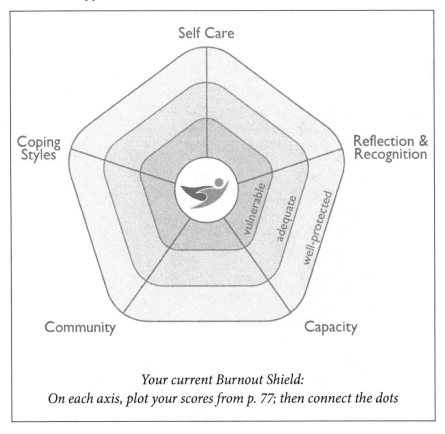

Your current Burnout Shield:
On each axis, plot your scores from p. 77; then connect the dots

Now it is your turn; follow the steps.

Voilà: you've created your Burnout Shield as it looks today!

Imagine yourself in the center of that map, and the Shield you draw around you represents how well you are protected from the stresses of your life and working environment.

What can you learn from looking at your Burnout Shield? Do any Key Areas stand out for you as being more protected? If so, congratulations! These are Areas where you want to keep doing what you're already doing. Do any Key Areas stand out for you as being least protected? You can use this result to guide you as to where (and perhaps in what order) you might choose to focus on making changes.

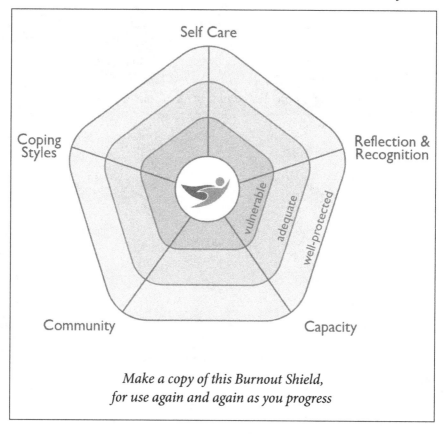

*Make a copy of this Burnout Shield,
for use again and again as you progress*

Use Your Burnout Shield Again and Again

Make a copy of your Burnout Shield that you can keep on your desk, in your pocket, or tucked in your wallet. Pull it out frequently to do a quick visual tour of the five Key Areas.

Also, whenever you feel the need to check your progress, you can also come back and re-score yourself on any or all of the Key Area Self-Tests. In the first year, you might want to review the Self-Tests as often as every six weeks. Keep track of how your scores change over time.

Remember: **Your scores on the Key Area Self-Tests are not judgments, just information.** Be gentle with yourself as you learn to:

- Value yourself
- Reflect; Recognize even small accomplishments
- Assess your load
- Ask for help
- Rethink your reactions

*Now, you're ready to go on to the next chapters,
which examine each of the five Burnout Shield Key Areas
in more depth. Read them in order, or skip to the Burnout
Shield Key Area you've identified as most important for your
focus right now. You're in control of your learning.*

Part III

Take Action

Chapter SIX

Self-Care: Are You Providing Your Body with the Basics that Keep It Going?

"I wish I could go back and tell myself that not only is there no trade-off between living a well-rounded life and high performance, performance is actually improved when our lives include time for renewal, wisdom, wonder and giving. [That would have saved me] a lot of unnecessary stress, burnout and exhaustion."
—*Arianna Huffington*

"In the event of an emergency, put on your own mask before assisting others."
—*Every flight attendant*

Self Care

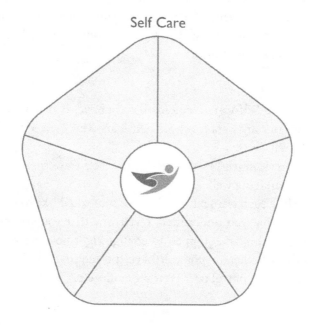

Elements of Self-Care

The following list includes elements of Self-Care. Despite these being some of the most basic functions of life, many of which we all learned to do in early childhood, it can be surprisingly easy to lose track of these elements as you focus on outside work or taking care of others.

Sleep	Exercise	Work/life separation	Compassion for self
Regular meals	Managing health issues	Time for personal needs	Healthy self-talk
Food choices (nutrients)	Time for personal life		

Overall Self-Care Goal

If you want to protect yourself from burnout, you need to provide yourself with the elements of Self-Care in your daily life. As you make changes, observe how you feel. Get to know your own needs and limits. Allow your needs to be a priority.

Where to Start

1. **Review** the Self-Care elements listed above. It may be helpful to review your answers from the Self-Care Key Area of the Burnout Shield Self-Tests.
2. Put a **check mark** by each element of Self-Care that you are currently managing well.
3. **Underline** each element of Self-Care that you'd like to improve.
4. Of those that you underlined, **circle** any that you are most motivated or feel most equipped to change right now. As you do this, consider whether or not you have the required skills, necessary resources, or control over your schedule, etc.

5. **Rebuild with positive changes.** Fill in the **To Do List** below with your plan for positive changes. *Note: You may want to wait to fill this out until after you've read the rest of the chapter.*

   Start where you have indicated you are the most motivated. We recommend that you start with one small change that is easy to incorporate into your daily schedule. Once you've been successful with that positive change, acknowledge your accomplishment and then continue to add more positive changes to your daily routine.

6. **Expand your insight, knowledge and skill level:** As you read on, you'll learn more about the different areas of Self-Care and how they impact your health and your ability to withstand burnout. We share some of our own stories and stories from the people that we've helped. You'll also find some additional resources and assessment tools that can help you become more familiar with aspects of Self-Care.

   Considering how vast these topics are, this chapter is intended only as a guide to some elements of Self-Care that are most directly related to your ability to withstand burnout. However, we encourage you to reach beyond this book. There are so many helpful Self-Care resources out there, and they can be the doorway to a great deal of healing of strength.

Positive Changes

Here are some examples of positive changes you can make for the different elements of Self-Care:

Sleep
- Sleep in a completely dark room.
- Go to sleep at the same time every night, wake up at the same time every morning.
- Avoid using screens (phone, computer, television) for an hour before bed.

Regular meals; Food choices
- Nutritious snacks — have them available when you need them.
- Eat more plant-based foods.
- Eat lunch in a different location than your desk.

Exercise
- Move your body more.
- Take the stairs instead of using the elevator.
- Walk around the building during a break or after lunch.

Managing health issues
- See a health care provider.
- Take the medicine/vitamins/supplements that you've been prescribed.
- Do 10 minutes of deep breathing every day (belly-expanding breaths that last 5 seconds in, 5 seconds out.)

Time for personal life; Work/life separation; Time for personal needs
- Do one thing every day that you enjoy.
- Take a vacation, even a short one.
- Give yourself a work email/text message curfew and stick to it.

Compassion for self; Healthy self-talk
- Be kind to yourself.
- Assure yourself that your needs are a priority.
- Allow yourself to experience feelings without judging them.

Self-Care To-Do List

Positive change I will try first:

_____

_____

_____

Positive changes I am interested to try in the near future:

_____

_____

Positive changes I may incorporate someday, but will put aside until I've successfully incorporated the changes listed above:

_____

_____

_____

Self-Care Results

Positive changes that have made the greatest difference in my life:

_____

_____

_____

Elements of Self-Care that I tend to let slip when I am under stress:

_____

_____

_____

Helpful Self-Care reminder for myself the next time I'm under stress:

_____

_____

_____

Get More Sleep

Are You Exhausted?

If you've ever thought, "I have no time for sleep." Or "I'll sleep when I'm dead," this section is for you. Stress from **lack of sleep is the "final straw" that puts many people over the edge from stressed-out to burned-out.**

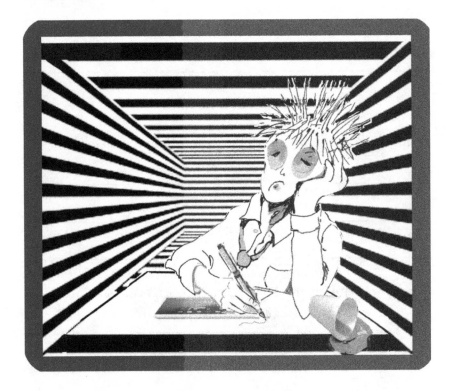

In this section, we'll focus on recovering from exhaustion and staying recovered.

One overall caveat. We have a warning to help you avoid a common negative feedback loop: **Beware of short-circuiting your recovery. As soon as you begin to feel more rested, you may feel so good that you are tempted to plunge right back into a pattern of over-productivity, once again skimping on sleep and rest. Don't do it.**

Beth: My (Lack of) Sleep Story

I knew there was a high risk of burnout in my field, but I thought my love for the work I was doing would keep me protected. In the early years of my nurse-midwifery career, on nights when loud beeps from my pager hauled me out of sleep at 3:00 a.m., I awoke with wild joy. I valued the honor and privilege of supporting women through the intimate journey of labor and birth, and I offered them every drop of my expertise and my commitment. Many, many hours later, after a good birth, I would tumble back into bed, weary but also exhilarated.

"If you love what you do, you'll never have to work a day in your life." This may be true, but don't be fooled. Loving your work isn't enough to protect you from burnout.

It may be that you love your work the way I did. When we are lucky enough to be able to do work that is fully aligned with our skills and talents, when we are privileged to make a true difference, such pleasure can make tolerating the pressures of our field seem easy. At least it can for a while.

My mistake was in believing that because I had such joy in my work, I could drop many of my other needs over the side. Ultimately, constantly dwelling in physical (and emotional) exhaustion killed that joy. Then work became just drudgery for me. I burned out.

I also shared in the health care field's culture of *machismo(a):* I took pride in believing I was tougher than the average bear. Although I tried to catch up on rest whenever I could, I never learned enough about sleep to create full recovery for myself. Instead, I was usually running on caffeine-drenched exhaustion.

As a result, after twenty-three years, when I finally did leave my field due to burnout, I had exposed myself to two decades of extremely random sleep cycles. After that, my body took a *full year* to re-learn how to let me sleep like a normal person. I had conditioned myself to "function" with random and inadequate sleep, and for a long time, random and inadequate sleep persisted, despite my exhaustion.

I now believe that professional education for careers in high-burnout industries should routinely include information about how to get enough sleep. Back when I was in grad school, I don't remember that anyone ever talked to me about making rest a priority. Maybe they thought it ought to be obvious.

It wasn't, not to me. But it *was* obvious to me that my midwifery professors at nursing school were pushing themselves to function on the same combination of coffee and sheer determination that eventually became my principal driver.

This experience finally drove me to learn much more about sleep, which I am now pleased to share with you. The basics appear here in this chapter. If sleep is a major challenge for you, you can find much more on our website, at www.burnout-solutions.com/sleep.

Fatigue and Exhaustion in Burnout

Fatigue, both physical and emotional, is the first major hallmark of burnout, and research suggests that lack of sleep can be a crucial stressor that can push a person over the line from being *stressed* all the way into being *burned out.*

This is one of the most important anti-burnout self-care skills: **Set a priority for rest and sleep. Back up that priority with stringent sleep habits.**

We believe teaching how to get enough sleep, especially in professions with irregular schedules, should be an essential part of a professional education.

How Much Sleep Do You Really Need?

Most people need **7 to 9 hours of sleep every night**.

By the way, you can't average it out. Seven to nine hours of sleep every night is *not* the same as 6 hours of sleep on weeknights plus sleeping in on weekend mornings. Trying to average out sleep is a recipe for accruing sleep debt, slowly but surely.

Sleep debt is the physical equivalent of spending more than you make. But in sleep debt, your interest payments and penalty fees can add up to burnout.

In sleep debt, your interest payments and penalty fees can add up to burnout.

There are consequences for missing just a little sleep. In fact, sleeping only six hours a night is considered "mild sleep deprivation." Studies by David Dinges at the University of Pennsylvania showed when well-rested volunteers went for one week on 6 hours of sleep each night, they suffered large decreases in cognitive performance (thinking) and alertness.

We're going to repeat this, because it's important. When these folks reduced their sleep for just *one week*, going from eight hours per night to six hours per night, they could not think as clearly, and they were unable to stay alert. It got even worse for them as time went on.

After two weeks of 6 hours of sleep each night, the volunteers' performance deteriorated even more: they were thinking and reacting *as if they had gone without sleep for 24 hours straight.*

Look at this equation. The impairment caused by two weeks of reduced sleep = the impairment of 24 hours without sleep. Even worse, other studies show the impairment from 24 hours without sleep = the impairment of being legally drunk. Conclusion: Reduced sleep for just two weeks can impair your performance as much as being legally drunk. **Reduced sleep can make you a danger to yourself and others.**

By the way, sleep deprivation affects more than just your performance. A 2013 study at the University of Texas also found that one week of getting just shy of six hours of sleep per night changed the functions of more than 700 genes, including genes that regulate inflammation and stress response.

Per the American Psychological Association, only one person in a thousand can function effectively on six or fewer hours of sleep per night.

The American Psychological Association, in its 2014 statement on sleep deprivation, said:

> ...over the long haul, perhaps one person in a thousand can function effectively on six or fewer hours of sleep per night. Many people who operate on chronic sleep debts end up napping during the day or fighting through long periods of sleepiness in the afternoon. Worse, most people who are sleep deprived do not even realize it. If you get sleepy during long meetings or long drives, chances are you are sleep deprived.

It is time to stop fooling yourself about your need for sleep. Recognize it as a necessity. Make it a priority.

But Some People Need a Lot Less Sleep, Right?

One scientific estimate says one percent of the population, or one in one hundred people, do seem genetically wired to need far less sleep than the rest of us. Other researchers' estimates are not as optimistic: they put that number at only one person in one thousand who truly needs very little sleep to perform well.

Given those odds — could *you* really be that genuine short sleeper? That one in one hundred — or even one in one thousand — who *truly* functions well on only 4 hours of sleep per night? Or are you like a much larger proportion of the population, who simply *thinks* they function just as well on a short amount of sleep?

Here's a simple test: if you consistently wake up feeling truly rested and refreshed after less than 7 hours of sleep, AND in quiet moments you don't find your eyes falling closed and your head dropping forward, you might be a true short sleeper.

On the other hand, if, despite feeling tired, you are somehow still able to push yourself to perform, you are very likely not getting enough sleep; you are probably fooling yourself about being a short sleeper. You are also likely creating safety hazards for yourself and others, and driving yourself further into burnout.

In that case, **it is time for you to stop pushing yourself and start making sleep a priority.**

Why Sleep?

What is the purpose of sleep?

Sleep recharges your brain. In order to recharge and maintain a finely tuned internal clock, which coordinates the timing and function of your sleep/wake cycle, metabolism, immunity, brain function and cardiovascular system, your brain needs regular intervals of light and dark.

During sleep, your brain also rebuilds its "battery" of glycogen, a storage form of fuel that your brain calls on at times of peak energy demand throughout the day. Peak energy demand for your brain includes such moments as: learning a new skill, solving problems in a crisis and using willpower.

Sleep builds long-term memory. Sleep is necessary for your brain to move short-term memories to long-term storage. With inadequate sleep, you are less likely to remember the facts, skills, events and people you need to recall.

Sleep empowers healthy emotions. Your brain uses sleep to replay emotions though your neurons in order to "file" them appropriately, as well as to put your day's emotions into perspective. When you deprive yourself of enough sleep, your emotional reactions while awake can become increasingly irritable and erratic.

Sleep rebuilds muscles. While you are awake and moving around, challenges to your strength and endurance create tiny rips in your muscle fibers, called "micro-tears." Sleep is necessary to repair these microscopic muscle-fiber wounds. This repair process is necessary to building stronger muscles.

Without sleep, your muscles cannot do as much of this repair; therefore, you don't benefit fully from your workouts. That is why professional coaches and athletes are acutely aware of the necessity for rest. Any athletic training regimen recommended by professionals will require plenty of sleep.

Sleep cleans up the "trash." Just as fire produces toxic by-products like smoke and ash, your body's healthy metabolism produces many toxins as by-products. While you sleep, your brain's neurons actually change their size and shape to allow circulation of fluids such as lymph that sweep that toxic build-up out of your brain and dispose of it. Sleep allows the brain to sweep away all that waste into the blood stream and lymph system, where it can be disposed of properly.

Sleep rebuilds your reaction time and judgment. For all the reasons listed above, a healthy and coordinated brain and body, which keep you and those around you safe, is one that has gotten enough sleep. As we will soon discuss in more detail, when you have not gotten enough sleep, you are at more risk for making errors, having accidents, and sustaining injuries.

In short, imagine your body as a grand hotel that houses your mind and spirit. Would you want to stay in a hotel with impaired institutional memory and staff that responded with irritable and erratic emotions, where routine maintenance is neglected and trash is left lying around? No? Then why would you operate your body this way? If you aren't getting enough sleep, your chronically exhausted body and brain lose essential services like these. Your functions can become poorly maintained, just like at that hotel.

Basic Anti-Burnout Sleep Rules

We assume you are reading this book because you want to recover, and stay recovered, from burnout. Here are our basic anti-burnout rules for recovering after a period of inadequate sleep:

1. Discipline your sleep schedule to get 7–9 hours of sleep on almost all nights.
2. Even adults need a bedtime ritual; create one or elaborate yours.
3. At first, also add *more* sleep time on nights and weekends, until you feel fully caught up. Then continue with your new routine of 7–9 hours of sleep each night.

Even Adults Need a Bedtime Ritual

Most parents learn that setting clear and consistent bedtime routines, tailored to each child, is necessary both for the child's wellbeing and for the parent's sanity. When activities are repeated the same way every night, putting on pajamas, brushing teeth and reading a bedtime story become a routine that helps the kids calm down and fall asleep.

Even though most kids look forward to the day when they'll be able to stay up as much as they want, it turns out that we as adults still need a set bedtime, and even a bedtime ritual, just about as much as kids do. However, as adults, we can give our bedtime routine the more scientific-sounding name of "sleep hygiene," complete with a list of rules of what to include and exclude from our pre-bedtime routine.

Really, though, whether you call it sleep hygiene, or your bedtime ritual, you likely still need it. For best function, our bodies crave consistency and order. In fact, repeating our earlier statement, in case you're skipping around: nearly all of us require 7–9 hours of sleep every night.

To allow ourselves to get all that sleep and to "shut down the brain" (as an engineer friend phrases it) each of us needs to build our "sleep drive." This is the body's internal clock that sets us up for sleep until it carries us off to dreamland. In order to keep this internal clock set correctly, we need to perform a set of actions pretty much in the same order, at about the same time every day.

Your routine may be slightly different than someone else's, but you'll function best if it is consistent for you. Just like two kids in the same family can need quite different routines to be able to settle down and go to sleep, the length and complexity of your personal bedtime ritual needs to be tailored to your own personality and metabolism.

Catch Up on Sleep. If at all possible, start your sleep plan with a week or two of restful vacation. **A Sleep Vacation's entire plan is simply that you catch up on sleep.** Turn off the alarm clock, darken the room, hang the "do not disturb" sign on the doorknob, and sleep, sleep, sleep. Help your loved ones to understand: you are doing this for them, too. True, you will be no fun for them on this vacation. But once you get rested you will have made a great start on being much better company for them.

Restorative Sleep. After you're initially caught up, discipline your sleep schedule to 10–12 hours per night — this means consistently going to bed way earlier than you are used to. It will take a while for your body to adjust to the new bedtime. Rebuild your bedtime routine to accommodate the new hours, and stick with it.

To add restorative sleep, also add 3–4 extra sleep hours to every weekend. Continue your extended sleep hours until you find that you are waking rested and refreshed, consistently and naturally, after 7–9 hours of sleep.

Discipline Your Schedule for 7–9 Hours of Sleep Nightly. Once you are waking refreshed, consistently and naturally, after 7–9 hours of sleep — NOW you can begin your regular sleep schedule. But to end burnout for good, you must continue to make your sleep and rest a top priority.

Rearrange your life so you get 7–9 hours of sleep every night, by following the Sleep Rules. This means you discipline your entire schedule around your sleep schedule.

Avoid Backsliding on Your Sleep. Watch out! There are two ways you can backslide.

First, it's very easy to simply let your sleep schedule become undisciplined, and end up in sleep debt again.

Second, once you start getting enough rest, you may feel so great that you fall back into habits of overwork. Be resolved that you will be protective of your sleep and not allow a few days or weeks of feeling good to derail you into burnout again.

When to Get Medical Help with Sleep

Many medical conditions can interfere with sleep. If this is true for you, you may need to address the medical condition directly. Or, if it's a chronic condition, you may need to get medical help from a sleep specialist. As we've discussed, people with burnout may not be as good about seeing a medical practitioner when they need to. Since you have resolved to no longer have burnout, consider these examples of situations where getting an appointment for health care is the right answer.

- Heartburn
- Snoring/Apnea
- Breathing problems
- Using sleep medications, and/or medications that interfere with sleep
- Insomnia
- Waking up at night
- Getting "enough" sleep, but still exhausted
- Pain
- Grief
- Anxiety or Panic
- Depression
- Medical conditions such as diabetes, thyroid conditions

Doctor's Orders: Kim's Story

In the first years of building her own website design business, Kim constantly felt big stress. Would her clients pay on time? Would revenue exceed expenses this month? When she was already working full-out to build websites for the clients she had, how would she find the time to recruit future clients? With all this stress, her health began to fall apart, and she certainly didn't have time for health problems.

Finally, in desperation, she talked to her doctor about more than just her current illness. She wanted to know about the *pattern* of illnesses she was experiencing. Her doctor —a great doctor—listened to Kim carefully and ran some tests. Finally, the doctor was ready to share her diagnosis. She simply said, "You are exhausted. You are going to have to create strict rules about your bedtime and follow every single one. This is something you will need to keep up for a matter of months. Check back with me in three months' time."

Kim relates, "At first, her recommendation really annoyed me. I am a grown woman; I get to go to bed when I want, right? Well, no, apparently, not at all." She goes on, "But it worked. After three months of my strict sleep routine, I had more energy and I was getting sick a whole lot less often. And I even got some bonus benefits: I could concentrate better and in the end, I was getting a whole lot more done."

Beth: Have You Got a Stunt Double?

I am a bit of a spoilsport at blockbuster movies, because while I watch them, I am never quite able to quiet at least three parts of my brain: the nurse, the mom and the responsible adult.

For example, take the final chase episode in the *Jason Bourne* series. During one of the movie's many intense and exciting getaways, one of the shadowy agents steals a huge black Hummer, which he drives at high speed in the wrong direction through freeway traffic. Pretty soon, he is actually ramming whole lines of civilian cars out of his way, hurling them off his speeding vehicle into a metal wake behind him.

Of course, part of me does enjoy the vicarious movie fun of shootouts and explosions, but as I munch my popcorn, I still wonder: if these events were real, who would have to pull the bodies out of all those cars, staff the emergency rooms, explain it all to the families, clean up the broken glass and tow the cars?

So why is it that in a movie, the consequences of extreme behavior are obvious to me, yet when I take a step back and look at my own real life, I can be so blind? How do I expect to be able to work at top speeds regardless of whether or not I've had any sleep, skipped meals, and ignored my own needs? Why aren't I more aware of the destruction caused by leading my own "blockbuster-style" lifestyle? In my mind, I'm working like a super-macho, high-performance action hero, but without sleep as a performance priority, I'm treating my body as if I had a stunt double.

I know I'm not alone in this. Many of us push ourselves this way, announcing, "Sleep is for wimps" and pushing ourselves ever harder.

But we don't have stunt doubles. We don't have teams of technicians to help us carefully craft each "close call," and we can't digitally erase any mistakes we make. We have one irreplaceable real-life body. (And if we are lucky, we also have a community of supportive colleagues, friends and family to help us when they can and a team of health care providers to help patch us back together when we get hurt.)

You Can Do It! You Can Get Enough Sleep

No more blockbuster living! Sleep deserves to be a priority in your life.

You need more sleep.

You deserve more sleep.

You are safer (and so are the people around you) when you get more sleep.

Best of all, you will feel much, much better when you get more sleep.

Your brain, your emotions, your health and your wellbeing will all function much better, when you get more sleep.

It is time to give yourself the gift of sleep. Track your results. You'll be amazed!

Low Blood Sugar and Your Brain's "Budgetary Shutdowns"

Do you know anyone who gets cranky when they are hungry? One of my patients called it being "hangry," a mix of being hungry and angry. There is a very good explanation for why this happens.

Your brain, like your car, only works when it has fuel. Your brain's fuel is your blood sugar. When you haven't eaten for a while and therefore your brain fuel is running extremely low, your brain, unlike your car, goes into survival mode and it chooses which sections of itself will get fuel and which sections will be temporarily shut down until more fuel can be found. That's right, your brain goes into budgetary shutdown mode.

Unsurprisingly, the most crucial section of your brain is the part that manages the basics of keeping you alive. It keeps your heart pumping, your lungs breathing, that sort of thing. This section also houses the emotionally reactive/survival part of your brain that behaves most like our animal predecessors. This part is especially good at fending off threats and fighting for survival. Rowr!

The section that your brain does *not* consider crucial for basic survival is the more-evolved reasoning and thinking part. When the entire brain is well-fueled and running efficiently, this part usually works to counterbalance the more aggressive tendencies of the emotionally reactive/survival part of your brain.

For instance: Say you are mildly hungry. You see food on a platter. Your animal/survival part of your brain says "MINE!" but the higher thinking/reasoning part of your brain says, "Wait just a moment. We are at a reception with the Queen of England. Surely, if we push her out of the way in order to claim the entire platter of food as our own, some very strong members of the Royal Guard will tackle us. That would hurt. Perhaps we should politely take just one and share the rest."

Look at that—you got what you needed but you did so in a socially appropriate manner. See how nicely those different parts of your brain interacted with one another when there was enough brain fuel to keep it all up and running?

However, when your brain goes into "hangry" mode, and the reasoning/thinking part of your brain has been deemed non-essential and is temporarily shut down due to budget cuts, there is nothing to counterbalance your emotionally reactive/survival part. This is the kind of situation that leads the "hangry" version of you to snarl at people. You snap, "Where the hell has this been?!" at Jeff from Accounting, when he is 15 minutes late with the budget report.

In that situation, if your brain had been completely up and running, the thinking/reasoning part would have recognized that Jeff's arm was in a cast and was probably slowing down his ability to type. But since this part of your brain was temporarily shut down, no reasoning was taking place. The only message that could come through was an unfiltered one focused solely on survival. The emotionally reactive/survival part was thinking, "Jeff, your late work threatened my ability to finish my presentation. If my presentation fails, I may lose my job. IF I LOSE MY JOB, I WON'T BE ABLE TO PROVIDE FOR MYSELF. JEFF, YOU THREATENED MY SURVIVAL!" Oh dear. Sounds like someone will be getting a visit from H.R. soon.

Blood Sugar Control: An Essential Aspect of Saving Yourself from Burnout

Beside a desire to avoid uncomfortable meetings with the H.R. department, blood sugar management is essential when you are saving yourself from burnout. In the big picture, extremely low blood sugar levels are just another form of stress. Every time you skip a meal, you are choosing to expose yourself to more stress, and your body already has more than it can handle. Your job is to minimize incoming stress as much as possible. Luckily, low blood sugar stress happens to be something that is completely within your control.

Another important aspect is that you really need your entire brain up and running in order to maintain healthy Reflection & Recognition practices. As you will read about in Chapter 7, the benefits that come from Reflection & Recognition are so powerful that we call them your "secret weapons" against burnout. The last thing you want to do is have a secret weapon that you can't use because it has been shut down due to budget cuts.

Keeping Your Brain Well Fueled

So, how do you keep your brain well-fueled with an even blood sugar level? Timing and food choices. You can maintain an even blood sugar level, and therefore a well-fueled brain, mostly with the timing of your meals and the foods you choose to eat. For people with metabolic issues such as diabetes, pre-diabetes and metabolic syndrome, they may also need medical help in getting their body to properly process food, but in any case, timing and choices are the main tools you have for balancing your blood sugar.

Meal Timing

You may find that in the beginning, when you are still burned out and not as able to handle stress, you will probably do better with frequent, smaller meals throughout the day. As your body gets healthier and your ability to deal with stress improves, your body will gradually be able to manage on larger, less frequent meals.

When most people are healthy, they need to eat at least three meals a day: breakfast, lunch and dinner. However, some people find they always do better on smaller, more frequent meals. There are even some people who do well on two large meals a day. Everyone is different. There is no right, no wrong, just what is best for you (as long as your blood sugar levels are healthy.)

The trick is to find what works for you and stick with it. Meal timing is all about planning ahead and getting into a routine. This doesn't mean you have to eat the same foods all the time, but you do need to get into a routine of *when* you will eat. Most importantly, you need to **have your next meal already planned *before* you get hungry.**

Going back to the car analogy, you never want your car to completely run out of gas before you refill it. It is best to refill your tank when there is at least a little bit left in there from the time before. If you wait until you run completely out of gas, you'll have problems.

Are you someone who has tended to skip meals in the past? As you work on getting into a meal routine, we recommend picking up some healthy snacks to have in your office, your bag or your car in case you fall into old habits and find yourself dangerously close to brain shut-down mode. A nice snack such as trail mix, yogurt or a protein bar can provide you with enough fuel to temporarily keep your entire brain up and running. You can use the time it buys you to reason and think about the best options for finding your next meal.

Food Choices

Your food choices can actually matter even more than your meal timing. This is because you can really mess yourself up by eating a "meal" that only provides you with a brief spike of blood sugar. Ultimately, you want your food choices to provide you with a good mix of complex carbohydrates, proteins and essential fats, because these foods provide a nice, steady source of blood sugar. In general, avoid sugar and other simple carbohydrates as stand-alone foods unless you are having a low blood sugar emergency and you are planning to have other food in the near future.

The goal here is to give you a general understanding of how these all work with relation to your blood sugar control, but I won't go into too many specifics about what to eat because there are literally hundreds of books available on this topic online or in your local library or bookstore.

As I describe how simple carbohydrates, complex carbohydrates, proteins and fats work in your body with regard to your blood sugar control, I ask you to visualize a campfire.

Imagine you are sitting by a campfire pit. It is a chilly evening, so the warmth you get from this fire needs to provide a nice, consistent source of heat to keep you warm for the next few hours.

In this blood sugar/campfire analogy:
- Simple carbohydrates (sugars, white rice, white flour) are like paper.
- Complex carbohydrates (fruits, vegetables, whole grains) are like kindling and small pieces of wood.
- Proteins (meat, eggs, nuts, beans) are like larger chopped pieces of wood.
- Fats (oils, nuts) are like big ol' logs.
- The heat from the fire is like the blood sugar level you will get from the food.

As you make your campfire, you notice that paper, when it is burned by itself, lights quickly and easily, but it only gives you a quick flash of heat and then leaves you cold again. The kindling starts to burn fairly easily and keeps burning and creating heat for a little while, certainly longer than paper did, but you need to put more kindling in there if you want it to keep burning for very long. The chopped pieces of wood take a while to start burning, but once they get going, they provide a nice amount of heat for a decent amount of time. Lastly, the logs are the most difficult to start burning, but once they do, they have the potential to produce a good amount of heat and burn the longest.

In the end, you find that the best campfire is usually built with a combination of kindling, some chopped pieces of wood and possibly a log or two if the fire burns hot enough. Similarly, a good blood-sugar balancing meal will have a mix of complex carbohydrates, proteins and healthy fats (from plants or fish).

Hopefully, this campfire analogy can also help you understand what happens when you have something sugary after you haven't eaten in a while. That sugary food, like the paper in the fire pit, burns quickly and makes your blood sugar spike up and quickly fall again. This can leave you feeling worse than you did before you had the snack. It is much better to choose foods that are a mix of complex carbohydrates and protein, and possibly even some healthy fats. Eating this blend of fuel sources will provide you with immediate energy as well as energy for the next few hours, until you are able to eat again.

A Note to Those Concerned about Weight Issues

I've known many patients who have gotten nervous when I started talking about eating more frequent meals or having snacks at the office. First of all, I totally respect any concerns you may have about weight gain or any desires you may have to lose weight. I hear you, I get it, I'm right there with you.

However, when it comes to the big picture, consider this: eating more regular meals will help you get your blood sugar levels under control. When your blood sugar levels are under control, your brain will work better. This means that you will be much more able to reason and make good food choices to get through the times of temptation that might have previously led you to break down and eat unhealthy snacks. It also means that having a brain that is working will also help you reset your internal clock, which will in turn help coordinate and maximize your metabolism.

Also, if you have made a habit of putting yourself through the stress of suffering through erratic highs and lows, eating sugary snacks and then starving yourself into low blood sugar levels, you may be throwing off the internal mechanics that help you efficiently process and metabolize your food. This can lead to problems like metabolic syndrome and Type II diabetes. I am telling you this to inform you, not scare you. Considering that the latest studies suggest that about half of American adults have either pre-diabetes or diabetes, this is important to know.

Your body and your brain work best when you provide it with consistent fuel. This is something that is completely under your control. On behalf of your body, I request that you please respect this responsibility and not make more problems for yourself. You've got enough stress to deal with! Please be patient with yourself and listen to your body as you go through this process. Ultimately, once your blood sugar levels have evened out, you will be in the best position, both physically and mentally, to keep your weight under control.

Regular Meals; Food Choices (Nutrients)

Eat More Plant Foods

When I was deep in burnout, I knew that eating a "rainbow" of fruits and vegetables every day would vastly improve my health, but it seemed too big a challenge.

Beth: My Burnout and Food Story

I used to have a "special" relationship with junk food. Have you ever been to the nurses' station or break room in a hospital? Grateful patients often gift their nurses with boxes of chocolates. The nurses bring in big rattling bags of salty-crunchy chips. Doctors and nurses who have kids in worthy organizations bring in the fund-raising candy bars and cookie dough.

Nurses know full well that junk food is really, really bad for our health and stamina. *This* nurse certainly knew it—I spent every clinic day counseling my pregnant patients on making healthy food choices. But while I spoke to them, I hoped they could not detect my guilty secret, which I suspected might be printed in large (but hopefully invisible) type, right there on my forehead: "I will be driving though some fast food place for dinner because there's no way I will have the time or energy to cook tonight!"

I did *buy* healthy food, but I rarely made time to *eat* it. Once, when talking about all the organic fruits and veggies I was buying, my husband commented that he was sure we had "the healthiest compost heap in the neighborhood."

Regarding junk food, night shifts were the worst for me. As a hospital-based nurse-midwife, my on-call shifts in labor and delivery lasted 24-hours. When I was up all night, my shift usually included that 3:00 a.m. moment when I found myself in the break room, gobbling up every bit of junk food I could reach.

I knew then that fatigue could create cravings for carbohydrates (sugars) and salt. I have since learned that making a series of decisions uses up your daily store of will power. Of course, on those 24-hour on-call days, making clinical decisions was a very big part of my job. So, by 3:00 a.m., there was no personal willpower left for me, just those intense cravings for carbs and salt. Gobble, gobble. Fast forward through many years of early-morning junk food binges at the nurses' station.

Finally, in desperation, I decided to walk my talk: every day, I decided to consume lots and lots and lots of different kinds of fruits and vegetables. I had to get creative in order to do that, though, since my old way of trying to eat healthy hadn't worked. I did it by adding a high-quality fruit and veggie concentrate to my diet that was backed by a lot of research.

Within about six weeks, I realized that every bit of junk food in the break room was no longer calling my name. I was walking right by it all, without even wondering if all those junky goodies on the break-room counter might be edible.

Another thing that astonished me: even though I was still tired (only sleep will cure sleep debt) I now had a good chance of waking up in the morning and feeling *good*. As with many new health habits, it takes time to realize you are seeing the benefits. But when I finally realized I was feeling *wellbeing,* my idiotic first thought was, "Hey, it's *true,* all the stuff I have been telling my patients about healthy eating, all those years!"

Of course it was true. I had been sharing the best research-based medical information with my patients: eating lots of fruits and vegetables ameliorates nearly every health challenge in the world.

However, in order to actually feel the benefits of fruit and veggie nutrition, you have to be eating quite a few of them, every day. And knowing something in your body and your heart is quite different from knowing it from academic research results. Experience and science, those two ways of knowing, had finally combined for me.

Another important benefit of eating all those fruits and veggies is prevention. But how do you feel the absence of a heart attack you will never have? That benefit may remain invisible.

However, prior to starting that fruit and veggie diet, one of my health challenges was having a puny immune system which seemed to meekly welcome every virus that came along. "A cold? The flu? Move right in and make yourself at home!" Many times a year I lost weeks of work due to viral illnesses.

Do you believe you have to be born with a "strong constitution" to have a healthy and strong immune system? In fact, much nutrition science shows that many people can build a robust immune system by eating a large variety of fruits and veggies every day.

I still love chocolate. But a brownie or candy bar has to be made of really exceptionally good ingredients for me to feel any desire to bite into it.

If your life is stressful, it can be life-changing for you to find some way to eat seven to nine servings of fruits and veggies daily. You'll feel better. You'll look better. People will notice!

Hindsight's 20:20. What I Learned about Nutrition and Self-Care

When I look back on that "simple" nutrition experience of mine, I realize I also learned many larger self-care lessons.

- Very occasionally, things that seem "too good to be true" actually *are* true. However, it's important to check their documentation carefully. **Beware of "proof" that is actually hype or hearsay.**
- **"Should" and "ought to" are lousy motivators.** For a while, I regularly told my patients they "ought to" be eating better. None of that produced much behavioral change.
- Before we leave the topic of "should," though: What *did* produce at least 9 months of positive behavioral change for most of my patients? Pretty much anything that they knew was good for

their babies. Eat healthy for themselves? Nah, too much work. Eat healthy *for the baby?* On it! In other words, **if you can find a personally compelling reason that your self-care will benefit someone you care about, then you are more likely to stick with it.**

- **Staying consistent with a small but powerful change can make a really big difference.**
- Even when you make that small but powerful change, it is so easy to get used to your "new normal" that you forget what life used to be like. You forget that you have indeed made a profound change for the better. Coming to believe the new normal has *always* been true for you is a common experience. Scientists call this *habituation.* It is a big reason why people don't stick to their new healthy changes, but drift back slowly to their old habits. They forget to notice what those new habits actually did for them. To avoid having your new healthy habit sabotaged by habituation, **keep track. Find a way to accurately compare the "old you" and "new you."**
- **Create several kinds of reminders to help you stay on track.** It's easy to get distracted from your goals. Create more than one kind of reminder. For example: Ask friends to (gently) remind you. Stick pictures or posters on your desk or your mirror. Place notes in your calendar. Add basic health habits to your daily "to do" list. Building a variety of reminders into your life provides important supports for healthy changes. Here's a reminder process that helps me: when I teach, I get reminded to walk my talk.

Physical Movement

Move the Body

Another way to shift your mood and recover your energy is through physical movement. Even a very little activity, such as 15 seconds of **dance moves** while sitting at your desk, can shift your mood. Wriggle your shoulders, wave your arms and smile. Boom, your mood may well have shifted into positive territory for at least the next few minutes. Let it be that simple.

Another idea: Have a **moving meeting**. The person you're meeting with may be as sick of sitting at a desk as you are. Why not take a walk together instead of sitting for coffee? If you need to take notes, you can record the meeting on your smart phone.

But exercise, real exercise, may have become a challenge for you, since you started heading into burnout territory. This can be especially true if you were never that good about exercise to begin with.

If you are an athlete now, despite your burnout, you have our admiration. After a quick warning of not pushing yourself too hard when you exercise, feel free to skip ahead.

But in terms of your real-life, burned-out experience, if exercise dropped out of your life some time ago, read on: this whole section on physical movement is for you.

These days, do you find it a challenge to think of exercise with positive anticipation? Perhaps you have been rolling through cycles of struggling to get yourself more fit, then getting injured and falling instantly back into your sedentary ways. Eventually, you notice, again, that when you sit all the time, everything hurts, and your energy slumps. So around the cycle you go again.

We've got some suggestions that will hopefully brighten the experience of moving the body, and make it much easier for you to stick with it and gradually, safely recover more and more of your fitness. The most surprising suggestion might be *pretending*, but we'll get to that in a minute. Basics first.

Be Safe. Rest First. Be Gradual

If you have burnout then you likely are — or were — a go-getter. Perhaps when you show up in an exercise class, or a stretching class, or even go out for a jog on your own, you have a tendency to push yourself and "go for it" the way you used to. When you work out in that frame of mind, you might try to do way too much. That is not likely to end well.

Also, when you are exhausted, the risk of injury from exercise goes way, way up. (For Beth, some small scars, the memory of innumerable sprained ankles, and even one formerly-broken wrist all attest to this risk.)

Let us rephrase this in a more positive light:

If you are truly exhausted, the priority is: ***Be safe: rest before exercise.***

Once you're at least somewhat rested, and your doctor says you are healthy enough for exercise, keep this in mind: **build your exercise**

tolerance gradually, at least initially. (If you choose to work with a trainer, get one who really understands your goals, your fitness level and the other demands in your life. If you are starting from burnout, having a trainer that pushes you hard is unwise.)

Monitoring your heart rate is helpful in avoiding overdoing it, while still ensuring that you are actually working out *enough*. Here's two ways to check your heart rate: you can **count your pulse** and compare it to the heart rate guidelines, or you can do the **talking/singing test**. Let's talk about both.

Count Your Pulse

The pulse check takes a few seconds of setup. You start by figuring out and writing down your maximum or upper limit heart rate for exercise.

And then (if you don't have a Fitbit or other heart rate monitor for instant feedback) you count your pulse for 6 seconds. (Compare the result of your 6-second pulse check to your target heart rate divided by 10. Easy peasy.)

1. **To figure out your "maximum" heart rate**: subtract your age from 220.
2. Aim to exercise between **50 to 70 percent of your maximum heart rate** most of the time.

For example:
- If you're 38 years old, your maximum heart rate is 220–38 = 182. Your target range is between 91–127 beats a minute.
  Or,
- If you're 59 years old, your maximum heart rate is 220–59 = 161. Your target range is between 80–112 beats a minute.

This is "moderate intensity" exercise. It is plenty to get your conditioning up.

NOTES: If you are exhausted, get some rest *first*. As an exercise beginner, or a re-beginner (your fitness is low *now*, even if you *used to* exercise regularly) use the 50% level as your moderate intensity heart rate for your exercise sessions at first (walking, swimming, whatever it is.)

For example:
- If you are 38 years old, and your heart rate max is therefore 182, and you are really out of shape when you begin, then your

beginning moderate intensity heart rate maximum (at 50%) is 91. (Your 6-second pulse check is 9.)

Or,

- If you are 59 years old, and your heart rate max is therefore 161, and you are really out of shape when you begin, then your *beginning* moderate intensity heart rate maximum (at 50%) is 80. (Your 6-second pulse check is 8.)

You may find these numbers reassuring. After a sedentary lifestyle, you will see that you do not need to push yourself hard to get a benefit. And, indeed, moving your body for 30 minutes a day, at the lowest heart rate level, and gradually, gradually increasing your moderate intensity heart rate target means that a) you are safer from accidents, b) you will be less likely to hate it and quit and c) you'll become less short of breath, your stamina will improve, your mind will clear and your body will ache less.

Use **gradual** as your most important watchword. By being consistent, you'll be able to *gradually* build up to working out at 70% of your heart rate maximum.

- **Add brief bursts — sixty seconds to 7 minutes — of high intensity exercise** to your fitness activity, and then drop back to the moderate intensity — until your heart rate is back to the moderate intensity level.

High intensity is defined as 70–85 per cent of your maximum heart rate. This is called **interval training.**

Going back to our examples:

- If you are 38 years old, your high-intensity burst of exercise will raise your heart rate to between 127 and 155. (Your 6-second pulse check is 12–15.)
- If you are 59 years old, your high-intensity burst of exercise will raise your heart rate to between 113 and 137. (Your 6-second pulse check is 11–13.)

Do the high-intensity level of movement for between sixty seconds and 7 minutes. Then do **active recovery: drop back to moderate intensity** movement for a while, until your heart rate and breathing have stabilized at your moderate intensity level.

Don't stand still when you drop back the intensity level, because moving builds your lung capacity. (And because you, too, are one of the cool exercise people. When we are walking slowly to calm our breathing back down, we cool exercise people call it "active recovery.")

Beth: Interval Training

I was thrilled to discover it. "Interval training" gave a dignified name to what I was doing anyway. Which was walking, mostly, and then occasionally staggering into a slow jog for a few feet until I was out of breath, and then dropping back to walking again, until I got my breath back. Interval training! This kind of exercise was *not* just me being super unfit and pathetic. This was me doing *interval training* (cue music: dum ta da dum!!) a powerful way to build greater fitness faster. Therefore, I am also one of the cool exercise people. And you can be one, too. Just add "interval training."

Interval training is actually more fun, too, because it adds a little more variety to your movement practice. And anything that adds fun makes it that much more likely you'll keep doing it.

The Talking / Singing Test

Don't have a Fitbit or other pulse monitor? Can't find your pulse? Hate all those numbers?

There's an even simpler answer.

If you are a little out of breath but you can still carry on a conversation while you're doing your exercise thing, then you're in the moderate intensity zone. If you can still sing, however, then it's time to increase the intensity just a little bit.

For a high-intensity interval training burst, push it up just until you reach a place where you can't talk except by gasping out a few phrases at a time. No higher. After the burst, go right back to your moderate intensity I-can-talk place, and keep moving at that level for a while. That's your active recovery mode.

Track Your Progress to Stay On Track

Having a way to track your movement activities is a powerful way to keep yourself at it, and to get back to it when you discover that somehow you've not done anything for a few days…or weeks.

There are innumerable ways to track your movement. Use the one that fits your budget and your style.

Tracker Options

- Paper tracking. Put hash marks on a calendar hanging on the wall. You see instantly where you stand.
- Cell phone movement monitor. Most newer cell phones have a program that will track your steps. On an iPhone, tap "Health" to access a step tracker. On Android phones, install "Google Fit."
- A fitness wristband, such as the Fitbit or Apple Watch or any of a number of competitors. These synch with your phone and desktop computer, and produce all kinds of nifty reports and graphs. Many also have options for tracking sleep, weight and both expended and consumed calories.
- An on-line tracker, like MapMyRun, which is free.

Would "Pretending" Make Exercise Fun for You?

What about the pretending we mentioned? Where the heck does that fit in?

Well, innumerable exercise manuals and fitness professionals will tell you that the best exercise for you is the one that you will actually do. And the one that you actually do is the one that you enjoy.

Beth: Making Exercise Fun

For a while, I was very confused by that advice about doing something you enjoy. I used to love ballroom dancing, running, and canoeing. Used to. So I tried Jazzercise and Zumba, because I thought they would be things I would love. I tried really hard to ignore and not compare myself to all the coordinated, happy, dancing people around me. I would just barely move to the beat, using small steps that kept me in MY moderate intensity heart rate range (which meant most of the instructor's dance moves and all of her jumping were right out.) But I couldn't maintain enjoyment when I found myself vigilantly monitoring my mood—to keep from being bummed out by what I couldn't do. It *would* have been fun for me, back when. I hope I will re-attain a fitness level where that kind of thing will become fun for me again.

But you know one example of something that worked really well for me? Pokemon GO. Yep, it's true. When it first came out, I would walk, even hurry-walk, many blocks out of my way to catch a rare Pokemon. On my walks, I frequently chatted with strangers who were delighted to share tips and information related to the game.

There are many other "pretending" games designed to get you moving. For instance, many of our friends love the app ZombieRun, which uses interval-training principles to get you moving to dodge zombies and run rescue missions for hapless imaginary "civilians" who are trapped by zombies. Our friends who love ZombieRun find themselves walking or running or biking a lot of extra miles every week, to complete those "missions."

Another, more complex pretending program is SuperBetter, found at SuperBetter.com. In this gaming system, you get to imagine yourself as a superhero (because, really, if you are one of our readers, you *are* a super-hero!) You also identify real-life "henchmen" and "sidekicks" who will help you meet your goals. SuperBetter might be excellent for you, if you would enjoy making parts of your real life into a story/game. Many people do.

PokemonGo, ZombieRun and SuperBetter are free, at their basic levels. You can have a lot of fun at those levels. And keep an eye out for new movement games; they are coming out all the time.

It is all about making it fun. If pretending makes it fun for you, then go for it. We'd love to hear what you find adds motivation and fun to your self-care activities.

Managing Health Issues

See a Doctor
Beth: Don't Ignore Warning Signs (Like I Did!)
Let's continue with the candid talk. Research tells us that many people suffering from burnout are less likely to see a doctor, or to seek help of any kind, for that matter. If this sounds familiar, don't feel badly. This could actually be due to the very nature of burnout itself. The third dimension of burnout, a lowered sense of personal accomplishment, can often leave people with an artificial feeling that it is hopeless to seek help or that they wouldn't be worthy of help even if they could find it.

In Chapter 8 I share my story of ending up on medical disability for a *full year* because I was too busy taking care of other people to stop and notice my own distress. However, before I got to that point, I ignored many of my body's distress signals, including frequent injuries and accidents. I sprained my ankle repeatedly, and even got into a serious T-bone motor vehicle accident at 2:00 a.m., when driving home from work while super-tired. On top of all that, I had social disasters such as falling asleep while sitting at the Thanksgiving table with family and friends. I also ignored family conversations that might have clued me in: my very young daughter told me that she never wanted to have children, because "Mommies are too tired."

Despite all that, I just kept on keeping on. My excuse? "My patients need me." But did they really need me to the point that I wouldn't be available to anyone anymore? Now I know: this is such a common behavior in burnout!

Interactive: Is It Time for You to Get Medical Help?

Medical issues can take you out of the game. They can seriously impair your ability to do your job, or to care for those you love. Check all the boxes that apply to your situation:

- ☐ Has it been more than a year since your last checkup? (Healthy people may not need to go for a checkup every year, but if you are having any health issues, including fatigue, you may not necessarily be considered healthy.)
- ☐ Have you got a chronic health issue that requires close monitoring to prevent serious complications, such as diabetes, asthma, lupus or high blood pressure?
- ☐ Are your symptoms increasing, perhaps pushing you to self-medicate or increase your other prescribed medications in order to help you keep going? (Examples: pain medicine, rescue inhaler, extra insulin, or medicine to help you sleep?)
- ☐ Are you finding you have increased your use of caffeine, sugary snacks or recreational substances, just to keep going?
- ☐ Are you having mishaps, accidents and injuries more frequently?
- ☐ Are your accidents or injuries getting more serious?
- ☐ Are you feeling depressed or anxious?
- ☐ Are people around you dropping hints that you don't look well or don't seem happy?

If you checked even one of these items, then yes, it is time to make and keep an appointment to see your health care provider. Did you check more than one? Then, like Beth and so many others, your "tough" stance is creating serious medical issues for you. You are overdue for some medical attention. Call for an appointment now.

Getting Medical Help for Your Burnout

If you need medical help to deal with your burnout, we urge you to seek it out. Due to the variable nature of burnout, there is no set protocol for treating burnout. From a billing standpoint, your insurance will likely not cover treatments if they are for a diagnosis of burnout alone. As the research in this area continues, policies change. Believe it or not, the medical recognition of burnout as a diagnosis differs from one country to another.

The United States used to be way behind other countries in the clinical recognition of burnout as a diagnosis. It is still not recognized in the US as a mental illness, however, as of October, 2015, the diagnosis coding guide (known as the ICD-10-CM) recognized "burn-out" under the code Z73.0: Problems related to life-management difficulty. It includes the symptoms of a state of both physical and emotional exhaustion.

Unfortunately, even though this is a step in the right direction, this is not a code that your doctor can use as a primary diagnosis for care. However, it can at least be listed as a contributing factor to one of your other diagnoses, and can help your care providers keep track of which medical treatments are the most helpful for you.

Health Care Resources for You

- For help with your emotional well-being, find out if your employer or your professional association has an Employee Assistance Program (EAP) in place. EAPs are confidential and are set up to help people get quick access to necessary services, often without any sort of out of pocket costs.
- Another resource for finding psychological help: http://locator.apa.org/.
- Do an internet search using the phrase "medical help resources <your state name>."
- If you are having urgent health problems, many areas have convenient walk-in or retail-center clinics and urgent care centers.
- If you want to try a different perspective on your health, consider health care providers other than conventional doctors (MDs). For example, nurse-practitioners, nurse-midwives, naturopathic physicians, chiropractors and acupuncturists are all types of licensed

practitioners that often offer more holistic care and longer appointment times, which give you more time to discuss your concerns (confirm this when you call to make the appointment.) All these types of provider groups also have excellent health outcome statistics. However, if your condition requires a medical specialist, see that specialist as well.

Burnout and Depression

There is no denying the strong relationship between burnout and depression. They are often found in the same person at the same time. Studies have found that depression can be diagnosed in anywhere from 50–90% of the participants who test positive for burnout. Some researchers argue that burnout is just one type of depression, but others argue that there is a distinct difference between the two. After working with so many clients and seeing how they respond, our impression is that it is important to distinguish between whether the person has depression by itself or has *both* depression and burnout.

This matters because treating depression that came about without burnout is different than treating depression that happened as a result of burnout. There are some treatments and therapies that will help regardless of whether or not there is a connection between the two, such as counseling methods like Dialectical Behavioral Therapy and Cognitive Behavior Therapy. But some of the medications that are used to treat depression may actually make someone with adrenal-burnout-related depression feel worse. In any case, it is important to get help if you are experiencing the symptoms of depression.

What Is Depression?

You may be depressed if you feel episodes of hopelessness, helplessness, and sadness, decreased interest in friends and things you used to enjoy, and cognitive changes such as pessimism and negative thoughts, especially about yourself. Less taking charge, more passivity. You can have distressing changes in your sleep patterns, your appetite, and even in your sexual drive. Depression can also bring in suicidal thoughts or thoughts about harming yourself. These last issues are critical and need to be addressed immediately.

Are You Having Trouble Finding a Reason to Keep Living?

Call now, don't wait. Or find the "click to chat" button at http://www. suicidepreventionlifeline.org/.

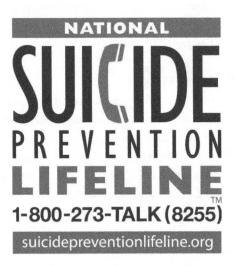

Mild to Moderate Depression

In mild to moderate depression, consistent self-care can sometimes bring relief:

- Exercise, even walking, can be as effective as depression medication, in some cases.
- Paying attention to your nutrition, especially whole food, plant-based nutrition. It turns out that plants have a tremendous number of nutrients that make our brains and our emotions work better, so eating more plant foods is good for your mental and emotional health, as well as your physical health.
- Address sleep issues. (Sleep deprivation makes both depression and burnout worse.)
- Connect with community and loved ones.
- If severe, or having suicidal thoughts — GET HELP.

Burnout and Severe Distress

If your burnout has you in deep distress, then know that *there is a way out*. We recovered, and you can too. You *can* win your way back to a more rewarding life.

Before you begin: Please give yourself some recognition — it took time for you to get into this deep place, and it will take a bit of time to get out. Be gentle with yourself. To climb up out of the pit is a "one step at a time, take it slow and easy" kind of process.

First things first. Please assess yourself. Have you had repeated injuries, or bad thoughts, that you brushed off as bad luck, on top of your burnout? This could be your body or your psyche, trying to get your attention with ever-louder emergency sirens.

Often, people with burnout have numbed their attention to their own physical and mental alarms. It's a known symptom of burnout. As they say... some people need to be hit over the head with a "brick" to get their attention. (Beth adds, "For me, it took a really BIG brick!") The good thing is, once you get the brick's message, you can stop the brick from hitting you so hard.

Take a moment to tune in to yourself. If any of these questions fit your situation, take action now:

- **Are you suicidal or do you self-harm?** Someone is always there to answer your call at The National Suicide Prevention Lifeline. Call 1-800-273-8255. *Call now.*

- **Do you fantasize about being sick or getting injured?** Some people who feel incredibly stuck in their situations may not actually want to die or cause themselves harm, but they find themselves fantasizing about these things as a way of mental escapism. Thoughts like "if I got into a car accident, it would be so nice because I would have to lie in a hospital bed and recover, and I wouldn't be able to work or take care of anyone else for weeks," can be actually comforting because in their current circumstance, it seems the only way imaginable to get a break. If you are feeling this way, it is very important for you to get help. You need an outside perspective. A counselor can work with you and help you find *actual* options for getting a break from your stressful situation that are far better than being broken and lying in a hospital bed.

- **Are you in pain?** Pain — both physical and emotional — can be a messenger that you need to stop what you're doing, or that you need to get help. But until it's addressed, pain is also an energy-sucking vampire. Get a diagnosis and get treatment. Depending on the nature of your pain, look for a mental health professional, pain clinic, or doctor/nurse-practitioner who comes well-recommended. Don't second-guess this one, get help. It may take a few tries to find the right practitioner for you, and the right treatment plan. Be persistent on your own behalf. (We know you are persistent, that's part of what got you into burnout, and it can get you out again, too.)

- **Are you frequently ill?** Get a diagnosis and a treatment plan. It may be that your burnout has caused a malfunction in your immune system or your ability to deal with stress. Or you may have an underlying medical condition — there are too many burnout-worsening medical conditions to begin to list them, and many are quite common. Get yourself to a well-recommended health professional who can sort this out for you. Likely, you will also need to make some other, non-medical changes as well — and that's where the Burnout Shield has a lot to offer. Give some of the techniques in this book a try! But first things first. Go get a diagnosis for any medical condition you may have, and follow your health care provider's treatment plan.)

- **Do you have PTSD?** PTSD treatment is an emerging area. See the Notes for this chapter for a link to a Mayo Clinic article which makes clear that much help is available to you now. Some vets with PTSD have also told us that the Burnout Shield process has offered practical strategies that help (though this is strictly anecdotal, so far.)

- **Do you have a history of trauma?** Trauma can have long-lasting effects on your moods and behaviors. If you have a past history of trauma and aren't sure if it is related to your current burnout or depression, it is worth exploring this with a mental health professional. There are many types of therapies that can help your brain process and recover from past trauma.

Time for Personal Life; Work/Life Separation

Interactive: What is Stopping You from Taking Your Vacation?

Check all the statements that apply to you:

- ☐ Work will pile up if I leave it.
- ☐ I am indispensable — they need me.
- ☐ While I'm gone, they may see I don't make a difference.

☐ It costs too much.
☐ I have lost my enthusiasm for travel.
☐ Nothing seems fun.
☐ Planning — yuck, no energy for that.
☐ Do I have travel, *again?*
☐ Last vacation, all I did was sleep.

These are all common burnout symptoms.

Americans Don't Take Enough Vacations

In 2014, nearly 42% of Americans did not take any vacation days at all. In 2016, 55% of Americans confessed to leaving vacation time unused.

Those statistics come from a widely-quoted pair of surveys done by Project: Time Off, and so does the table below. Can you relate to any of these reasons for not going on vacation?

	2014 Overwhelmed America	State of American Vacation 2016
Return to a mountain of work	40%	37%
No one else can do the job	35%	30%
I cannot financially afford a vacation	33%	30%
Taking time off is harder as you grow in the company	33%	28%
Want to show complete dedication	28%	22%
Don't want to be seen as replaceable	22%	19%

Table 6.1 Reasons Vacation Time Is Left Unused

In addition, Project: Time Off wrote this: "Real workplace change depends on America's managers. To workers, the boss is the most powerful influencer when it comes to taking time off, even slightly more influential than the employee's family (24% put the boss as number one, 23% said family.) In fact, **80 percent of employees said if they felt fully**

supported and encouraged by their boss, they would be likely to take more time off."

Can you relate to that statement, as well? In many lines of work, your boss may never get around to saying, "Have you put in for your vacation time?" If you own your own business, you may get paid only when you work. So being your own boss can be tough, too, when it comes to taking vacations.

Either way, consider this: you may be most trapped by your own mindset. While burnout would be far less of an issue (and productivity would rise!) if all employers took care of their employees the way they should, *we can't wait for that to happen*. We need to learn to take care of ourselves. Even in tough situations.

What would happen if you decide that your own welfare is important enough to take, and use well, the rest and relaxation time to which you are entitled?

Take Breaks for Personal Needs

"I'm often too busy even to use the bathroom."

Let's be a little frank, here. There are not many statistics on which professions are too busy to have time to pee. Even less is known about those that don't have time to poop. But as health care providers, we know this is a very common issue with our patients and people in our profession. We also know how often this topic gets publicly ridiculed, which doesn't help.

Consider the plights of nurses and teachers. Hospital nurses often run their legs off throughout every shift, each nurse caring for 4–8 severely-ill patients. K-12 teachers often find themselves alone in a classroom of 25, 30 or even 50 children. With these charges, nurses and teachers find very few opportunities to go off to a bathroom during their workdays. (In fact, in medicine, one name for a painfully stretched, overfull bladder is "nurse's bladder," but the problem is by no means restricted to nurses.)

Doctors have similar issues. For instance, we heard from an optometrist in private practice in a clinic in one of those big-box stores: "They book my patients very close together and I am always hustling to try to stay on time. When I am running at all behind schedule, and I take a moment to rush to the restroom (which, in my office suite, is just off the waiting room) I get glared at by every patient there. It's very uncomfortable!"

Sometimes there is more than just social pressure not to take a bathroom break. A report by the humanitarian group Oxfam America revealed that in the poultry processing industry, workers are often flat-out denied the opportunity to take a bathroom break by their managers. In their report, they note that this practice had become so intense that workers often suffered as they turned to extremes such as urinating themselves or wearing diapers, and they often reduced their own fluid intake and suffered higher rates of bladder and urinary tract infections.

Even children in many public schools have issues with not being able to use the bathroom when they need to. This is related to having to ask permission (and sometimes being asked to wait) as well as dirty bathrooms and bullying that occurs while they are in the bathrooms. We even found a study titled "Do public schools teach voiding dysfunction?" which concluded: yes, yes, they do.

From our experience, here's our list — probably incomplete — of folks who are deterred from using the bathroom as often as they need to:

- Nurses
- Doctors in office practices
- Poultry processing workers
- Many (most?) other health care professionals
- K-12 teachers
- Parents of small children
- Children in some public schools
- Office workers
- Factory workers
- Retail workers
- Customer service workers
- People who are the "wrong" gender for the available restrooms

From a burnout perspective, why is this problem worthy of having its own section? Three reasons:

First, **ignoring your own needs is a classic issue for people who are burned out, or on their way to being burned out.** Either you may be in a high-stress work environment where you don't have control over one of the most basic functions of your body, or you may be used to ignoring your body's basic signals. This can often be a symptom of tuning out a number of other important messages from your body and brain about your health status.

Second, there are some serious **health risks**. Frequently holding your pee for too long can create an increased risk of bladder infections (which can, in turn, lead to kidney infections).

Not pooping often enough can lead to constipation, which is uncomfortable, and may risk further health complications as well. These complications can include things like hemorrhoids, fissures and other problems that can make it especially difficult to sit through a day of work.

Third, if you're routinely not able to urinate when you need to, then you're likely compensating by not drinking nearly enough fluids, especially water. Yet, **drinking lots of water is necessary for thinking clearly, managing your healthy moods, reducing your risk of bladder infections, avoiding constipation and controlling overeating** — among a host of other benefits.

There is a lot more you can learn when it comes to healthy personal habits. To add some fun by switching to a more game-based way of learning, check out Appendix B.

Compassion for Self; Healthy Self-Talk

Thoughts on Self-Care:
Why Does Helping Others HAVE to Include Helping Yourself?

Most people enjoy helping others. Some of us have a passion for helping others.

People who feel this way often feel obligated to make the world a better place, no matter what. We're usually aware that we run a higher risk of burnout in dedicating our lives to this passion, especially if we work in one of the "helping professions." There are many people in this world who need so many different kinds of help!

Yet we're pretty sure *we* won't burn out, because helping others is a virtue, and we are very virtuous. Also, we love helping others. It really is a joy.

But. Now, perhaps, here you are, burned out, or nearly so. Wanting to help others but running out of emotional and physical energy.

What is a basic requirement for helping others? Being available, not being burned out. See what I did there?

The truth is, your body and your psyche will do the best they can to defend you against a situation that is *all give and no receive*. If you have no rejuvenating strategy in place, then one day you can wake up and all the joy of giving has drained away. You can find that you're emotionally exhausted, cranky and maybe you've even become cynical. At that point, maybe you are super tough and super determined. Maybe you ignore all those cues, too. So, like Beth, maybe you end up in big health trouble, maybe even in the hospital.

We each learned this the very hard way: "Taking care of myself is *required* for me to be good at caring for others." To put it another way, the people I am caring for *need* me to take care of myself.

If you are one of those with a passion for helping others, this is the secret that makes taking care of yourself into a virtue: *I practice self-care because I have to in order to be able to continue caring for others. I am valuable. I matter.*

Chapter SEVEN

Reflection & Recognition: Engage Your Brain's Most Powerful Reward Circuits

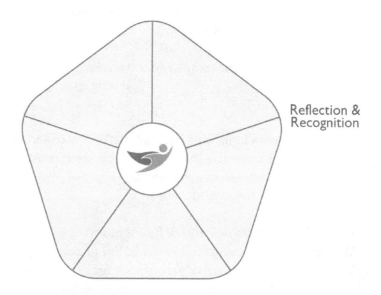

Reflection & Recognition

"And time for reflection with colleagues is for me a lifesaver; it is not just a nice thing to do if you have the time. It is the only way you can survive."

—*Margaret J. Wheatley*

Quick check in:

Have you been acting from a reactive state of mind or a reflective one? How frequently do you reflect on what is meaningful to you and acknowledge your own accomplishments?

Elements of Reflection & Recognition

The list below includes elements of Reflection & Recognition. As you've probably noticed, a lot of these things have to do with your internal thought processes and patterns. If it seems like this area is just "touchy-feely fluff," *don't be fooled!* This section is the most helpful for resetting your brain back to Reflective as the default mode, as we discussed in Chapter 2.

Engagement in work	Recognition type	Achievable goals	Awareness of injuries
Daily reflection	Recognition by others	Self-awareness	Spiritual-type practice
Meaning of life	Self-recognition	Acceptance of feelings	

When it comes to fighting burnout, Reflection & Recognition skills are your secret weapons. Thankfully, if you are exhausted, this is the area where the main activity is *thinking.* Some of your smallest efforts can have the greatest rewards.

Overall Goal in Reflection & Recognition

Your mind is the first and most powerful line of defense against burnout. When you use the Reflective part of your brain to deal with incoming feelings or solve problems, you have more endurance, the pain you experience is less intense and lasts for a shorter amount of time. You also have more control over your emotions, are better able to reason, and have a greater ability for creative problem solving. For most people, it takes frequent, repeated practice using the reflective aspects of your mind to reset the Reflective mode as your "default" setting rather than the Reactive one.

Similarly, with a few changes in the Recognition area, you can engage your brain's most powerful reward circuits in order to improve your engagement and motivation in ways that work for *you.*

Where to Start

Self-Awareness; Awareness of injuries; Acceptance of feelings
- Sit quietly for one minute. Notice your breathing, notice how your body feels in the chair and how your feet feel against the floor. Is your breathing quick and shallow or slow and deep? Are your shoulders relaxed? Are your feet in a comfortable position?
- If you feel pain or tension, ask yourself, "Do I need to be doing this activity right now?"
- If you experience an unpleasant feeling or emotion, pause and take note of it without judging it as good or bad. If you are ready for a next step, think back about the events or thoughts that led up to that feeling or emotion.

Daily reflection; Engagement in work
- Keep a daily reflection journal.
- Put a note on your bathroom mirror to remind you to do a daily reflection.
- Think back: What was your inspiration for going into your current career?

Meaning of life
- Check in with yourself—what are your core values?
- At least once a day, do something that is meaningful.
- Find a community of people who share your values.

Spiritual-type practice
- Make time to practice your religious or spiritual practice (if you have one.)
- If you are curious, look into different religious or spiritual groups in your area.
- Connect with your religious or spiritual community (if you have one.)
- Get out into nature whenever you can.

Self-Recognition; Achievable goals
- Identify small ways you can celebrate your own accomplishments.
- Break large goals into a chain of smaller, more achievable goals.

- Create a visible way of recognizing when you achieve your goals, including sub-goals.

Recognition type; Recognition by others
- Identify your own preferred recognition type (see later in this chapter.)
- Share your preferred recognition type with your supervisor.
- Start recognizing achievements with others around you. Use a symbol, a catch phrase, a high-five or some other ritual to help you recognize achievements.

Reflection & Recognition To-Do List

Positive change I will try first:

_____

_____

_____

Positive changes I am interested to try in the near future:

_____

_____

_____

Positive changes I may incorporate someday, but will put aside until I've successfully incorporated the changes listed above:

_____

_____

_____

Reflection & Recognition Results

Positive changes that have made the greatest difference in my life:

_____

_____

_____

Elements of Reflection & Recognition that I tend to let slip when I am under stress:

_____

_____

_____

Helpful Reflection & Recognition reminder for myself the next time I'm under stress:

_____

_____

_____

Marnie: Brain Function and Mindfulness

One of my first "Aha!" moments about burnout came when I read an article by Judy Willis MD. (We've reprinted selections from her article here with permission.) Dr. Judy Willis, a board-certified neurologist in Santa Barbara, California, has combined her 15 years as a practicing adult and child neurologist with her teacher education training and years of classroom experience.

She originally wrote this article for teachers, encouraging them that feelings of burnout are *not* a reflection of their teaching skills. Her explanation of what had happened to our burned out brains made so much sense. I felt reassured!

Reading her article was the first time I actually felt confident that I could recover from burnout. It was like I had been shown the secret code behind how burnout happened. I felt like Morpheus in the movie *The Matrix*; as I looked around me, everything looked different. I could see how some things would lead to burnout and others would help protect against it. I was no longer defenseless.

If You're Burned Out, Your Brain Has Rewired to Survival Mode

(From *How to Rewire Your Burned-Out Brain: Tips from a Neurologist,* by Judy Willis, MD.)

> What I offer from the nexus of my dual careers as a neurologist and classroom teacher are interpretations and correlations from the neuroscience research to teaching and learning. Neuroimaging studies reveal the metabolic changes in regions of the brain where activity increases or decreases in response to emotional or sensory input.
>
> There are specific and reproducible patterns of changing neural activity and brain structures associated with stress. In the high-stress state, subject's scans reveal less activity in the higher, *reflective* brain and more activity in the lower, *reactive* brain that directs involuntary behaviors and emotional responses. Prolonged stress correlates with structural increases in the density and speed of the neuron-to-neuron connections in the emotion-driven reactive networks of the lower brain, and corresponding decreased connections in prefrontal cortex conscious control centers.
>
> The explanation of these changes is generally attributed to the brain's neuroplasticity of "neurons that fire together, wire together." The brain literally rewires to be more efficient in conducting information through the circuits that are most frequently activated.
>
> As you internalize your thwarted efforts to achieve your goals and interpret them as personal failure, your self-doubt and stress activate and strengthen your brain's involuntary, reactive

neural networks. As these circuits become the automatic go-to networks, the brain is less successful in problem-solving and emotional control. When problems arise that previously would have been evaluated by the higher brain's reasoning, the dominant networks in the lower brain usurp control.

Reset Your Brain's Default Neural Network from Retreat to IGNITE!

The good news is that you can apply what you now understand about your brain's survival mode to take back voluntary control of your choices. You can activate the same neuroplasticity that gave dominance to the lower brain networks in the burnout state to construct a new, stronger default response. With more successful experiences achieving goals, you can reset the circuits that will direct your brain to access its highest cognitive resources for creative problem-solving. You can build up new, improved circuitry, switching your responses from retreat to IGNITE!

Since a repeated pattern of effort-failure set up the brain's survival response to withhold effort, you'll need to strengthen the pattern of *effort toward goals can result in success.* Your weapon of mass reconstruction can come from your brain's very powerful drive for its own neurochemistry—dopamine and the pleasure it brings.

The plan to guide you comes from the video game *model* that works because of three components: buy-in, achievable challenges, and frequent awareness of incremental progress en route to the final goal.

The fuel that motivates the brain to persevere through increasing challenge, even through failed attempts, is *dopamine.* This neurochemical produces the pleasure of intrinsic satisfaction, and increases motivation, curiosity, perseverance and memory. Dopamine is released when the brain makes a prediction or achieves a challenge and gets the feedback that it was correct. This can be in situations from the "Ah, I get it!" of figuring out a joke to the satisfaction of completing a marathon.

Just as the video game model can be applied to building a

growth mindset in students, the same model can help rewire your mindset regarding your ability to achieve teaching goals at school. As in the video game model, to get the dopamine-pleasure response from challenges achieved, you'll need to plan for your brain to experience *frequent* recognition feedback of *incremental progress*. You should set your "rewiring" goals by their desirability and by the goals' suitability to be broken down into clear segments. This way, you can chart your goal progress as you achieve each stepwise challenge. The pleasure burst of intrinsic motivation that will accompany your recognition of each progressive increment achieved in the goal pathway will keep your brain motivated to persevere.

Goal: Buy-In for Your Brain's Neural REWIRING

Buy-in and relevance are important in choosing your rewiring goal. Since your goal is to rewire your brain's expectations that your efforts will yield progress, even through increasing challenge, you need to really want the goal. This is not the time to challenge yourself with something you feel you should do but won't really look forward to doing, such as dieting, climbing stadium stairs, or flossing after every meal. Select a goal that you would enjoy en route and at the finish.

Usually goals are tangible. Some are visible, such as planting a garden or making pottery on a wheel. Others are auditory, such as playing an instrument, or physical, such as learning tai chi. But your goal can also be the increased amount of time you sustain an activity such as journaling, practicing yoga or sketching.

Your Rewired Brain's Default Changes
from Defeat to Ignite

As you meet your incremental goals and have repeated experiences of dopamine-reward, you will literally change your brain's circuitry. Repeated effort-reward experiences promote neuroplasticity, and this makes a neural network that *expects positive outcomes* into your new default network. This is because your "rewiring" goals helped your brain build stronger and more connections into a memory pattern where effort brings pleasure.

As with other networks not used, the previous lower brain stress-activated go-to response network you developed, the one that caused you to *react to problems*, will be pruned away from disuse.

You'll be rewired with optimism and renew your positive expectations. With your higher, reflective brain back in control, you'll be able to access your perseverance, innovation and creative problem solving when you return to the classroom.

Just be sure you take time to recognize each small success and creative problem-solving opportunity. Keep up the habit of breaking down big challenges into opportunities for recognizing incremental progress and receiving your well-deserved dopamine reward. The brain needs that battery recharge to sustain the positive expectations that motivate continued effort—so that you can stay engaged and move to the next step toward your teaching goals.

There's No Time Like the Present

When people are distracted, accidents tend to happen. This is such a universal occurrence that movies and television use "accidental slip-ups" to illustrate when a character's mind is elsewhere. The girl who is thinking about that boy she just met accidentally misses the mug when she pours her coffee. The boy who is worried about his big presentation accidentally bumps into someone and drops all his important papers. We all know what it means when we see these kinds of mistakes — that person's mind is elsewhere.

For those of you who have much more important responsibilities on a day-to-day basis, your mistakes and accidents can have more serious implications than spilled coffee or dropped papers. Your life is filled with important elements, and these elements deserve your attention, but not at the cost of your safety. If you aren't downright purposeful about staying focused in the present, you risk having your own "accidental slip-ups."

The skills required for this kind of purposeful presence of mind may not come naturally to you, but they can be developed. The practice of mindfulness or mindfulness meditation provides a fairly approachable method of developing these skills.

Researchers have found that workers trained in mindfulness improve their workplace safety and efficiency rates and workplace satisfaction scores. It has been so effective that mindfulness is starting to be incorporated into workplace safety training throughout many different industries around the globe, and not just in the human service industries. For example, the oil shipping company Alaska Tanker Company has used mindfulness training as an integral part of their innovative workplace safety training for merchant marines and shore staff. Their resulting safety record has broken industry records, winning them widespread recognition and awards.

Marnie: Shrugging Off Barriers to Success

Mindfulness training is one of the most powerful methods for combating burnout, and it was one I almost missed out on completely. I must admit, being raised a Midwest girl, I was initially turned off by some of the language that is commonly used in mindfulness. I didn't think a salt-of-the-earth, nose to the grindstone, put your head down and power-through person could get anything useful from being told to be "non-judgmental" and "in the moment." I was someone who skated to where the puck was going to be! (That's a Gretzky ice hockey reference, for those of you who aren't familiar.) It was all about pushing forward and anticipating what was next.

However, I hadn't realized what a huge part of the equation I was missing by not *also* being in the moment. What better way to anticipate where the puck is going to be than by knowing exactly where it is right now? And how do I expect to be able to push myself as hard as possible without breaking myself, if I don't know how close I am to that breaking point in each moment?

Mindfulness also helped me get past my curse of the "should." I used to spend a lot of time and energy thinking about what I *should* have been feeling and what I *should* have been doing, rather than what I actually *was* feeling and doing. This "should" version of me was a huge distraction. I had thought it was a goal-setting exercise, helping me to aspire to be even better than I was, but as it turns out, it was a barrier to my success.

The "Should Suit"

To teach this concept to my patients and students, I call it the "should suit." Let's say you try on a jumpsuit that is in your size, but it doesn't fit. You double check the size, put it back on and think, "Well, it *should* fit, it *should* be comfortable," but all the while the sleeves are too short, the pants are too tight, and the whole ill-fitting suit is limiting your movement. The people around you might even be saying that it *should* fit you and *should* feel just fine, but it doesn't! No matter what, the more you ignore how you *actually* feel, the more it slowly forms the worst wedgie you've ever had.

In the same way, if you are only thinking about what you *should* feel, you aren't doing yourself any favors. What matters most is how you *actually* feel. This is the most valuable information. If you can observe your feelings as they actually are, pleasant or unpleasant, you can learn a lot about what you actually need. You can also learn how to best proceed toward your goals, no matter what they are.

For me, mindfulness training was the missing link when it came to my burnout protection.

Mindfulness

Mindfulness is a method of concentrating your calm attention on all the features of the present moment, including your own feelings and sensations. This kind of awareness without being defensive or reactive is often described as *witnessing*, or *being present in the moment.*

In other words, mindfulness is a way of training your brain to use the Reflective default mode.

As we've already discussed in Chapter 2, when you are solving problems or confronting difficulties using your brain's Reflective mode, you are using the part of your brain for the greatest capacity for a productive outcome. When in this mode, you have more endurance, while pain you experience is less intense and lasts for a shorter amount of time. You also have more control over your emotions, are better able to reason, and have a greater ability for creative problem solving.

For many of us, our work involves "emotional labor." That is, we often face emotionally-charged encounters and need to manage our emotions as part of our job. When we experience emotional labor while our brain is in the Reactive mode, we are likely to fall into emotional exhaustion (the first dimension of burnout.) Emotional exhaustion is especially likely if our work requires us to display false cheerfulness, also known as "surface acting."

Thankfully, research has shown that mindfulness skills, especially when consistently practiced, reduce both surface acting and emotional exhaustion. This is because people who are consistently practicing mindfulness are able to calmly and effectively respond to problems as they arise. Mindfulness training teaches people to simply notice and observe those feelings without feeling compelled to either repress them or act on them.

Multiple Levels of Mindfulness

There are multiple levels of mindfulness; research shows that they can be beneficial in reducing burnout and improving productivity.

At the initial level of mindfulness, you simply find yourself paying more attention to sensations and events in and around you from moment-to-moment. Indeed, some people tend to be naturally mindful in this way. Others of us need to remind ourselves to stay attentive to the present moment in a way that "casts a wide attentional net," without multitasking, ruminating, or being hampered by the emotional baggage we might otherwise attach to events.

The ability to identify and label your feelings is key. There is a real therapeutic value to this practice which can even be seen in brain scans. The scans of people who are sitting in silence and "simply observing and labeling negative emotions," show that observing negative emotions and labeling them calm the emotional center of the brain that would otherwise be defensive or reactive.

As an example of this first level of mindfulness, a study of extremely busy servers working in seven restaurant chains found that servers were rated as more productive by their supervisors if they managed to "situate their minds in present moment time despite psychological pressures to the contrary." In other words, these servers stayed attentive, instead of getting caught up in "automatic thought or behavior patterns." The researchers studied this industry because servers in these high-pressure environments must constantly respond to changing conditions and demands.

Another study showed that mindfulness skills can even impact how qualified you seem to be to do your job. In this study, absent-minded or non-emotionally present supervisors were perceived as disrespectful and incompetent. On the other hand, employees whose supervisors were more mindful felt valued and treated with respect. These employees were also more satisfied with their jobs.

At a deeper level of mindfulness, you train your mind to stay more deeply and consistently in Reflective mode by doing daily mindfulness meditations and mindfulness exercises. The goal is not so much to attain rest and comfort, as in other meditation practices. Instead, mindfulness mediation is aimed at creating a state of *noticing without judgment.* This mindfulness state allows you to stay alert as your feelings, emotions and observations arise and dissolve.

You develop these skills by constantly retrieving your mind from distracting memories, thoughts of judgment, speculation or other non-present-moment thoughts or feelings. In mindfulness mediation, this kind of attention is practiced while you are in stillness. In mindfulness exercises, this kind of attention is practiced while you are active. The more you practice, in both modes, the more your brain stays in Reflective mode.

For some additional thoughts on mindfulness, we turned to our colleague, Dr. Donielle Wilson, ND, who specializes in stress reduction.

What Is the Difference between Mindfulness and Meditation?

(With thanks to Dr. Donielle Wilson, N.D., for allowing us to reprint this from her website, https://doctordoni.com/2016/09/how-mindfulness-and-meditation-decrease-stress/.)

Mindfulness is actually a type of meditation. Jon Kabat-Zinn says that, "Mindfulness means paying attention in a particular way; on purpose, in the present moment, and non-judgmentally."

Meditation in various forms, including transcendental meditation, induces a type of brain activity that is different than being alert or being asleep. It is actually 2 to 5 times more relaxing and restful than sleep and it is this deep state of relaxation which allows the body to heal from stress and, because it involves both sides of your brain, it helps build the communication pathways between the logical left brain and the creative right brain.

How to Start Meditating or Practicing Mindfulness

Meditation is often represented as sitting still, cross-legged on the floor, with your eyes closed. That is certainly one way to meditate, but it is also possible to meditate or practice mindfulness while sitting in a chair or doing activities such as walking, doing the dishes, brushing your teeth, eating, or showering.

Another form of mindfulness is biofeedback, which involves focusing your attention on your body to change your blood pressure or heart-rate variability. Personally, I like to practice mindfulness while taking care of our rescue cats and while taking our dog, Aphrodite, for a walk.

A simple way to get started is to put your focus on just one thing. For example, you could put all your focus on the word "one." Or you could put your focus on your breath—inhale slowly, exhale slowly, and repeat, noticing how each breath feels. Or you could focus on a "mantra"—a positive affirmation or thought, similar to a prayer.

Whatever you choose to focus on, each time you notice that your mind has wandered to another thought (and it will), quietly and calmly bring your attention back to that one thing. You could spend as little as 5 minutes or as long as an hour, or even several hours, practicing mindfulness.

During my first MBSR class we started by eating a raisin in a mindful way. We first picked up the raisin and looked at it. Then we felt it and smelled it. Finally, we put the raisin in our mouth, at first not biting into it, and then noticing how it tastes when we did bite into it. We chewed it at least ten times before swallowing it. A raisin never tasted so good! You could try this (as long as you are okay eating a raisin) as a way to start experiencing mindfulness.

If you'd like to develop your mindfulness skills further, look for an experienced, well-trained teacher. Participants in mindfulness programs that last 5–8 weeks have been shown to maintain a decreased level of emotional exhaustion up to three months later. Continued mindfulness practices and periodic refresher classes further maintain and boost the benefits. (Note that, while "stress reduction classes" are often helpful in other ways, not all such classes teach mindfulness.)

- Join a class or online course that teaches mindfulness meditation, which might also be called "Vipassana" meditation, or "witness consciousness." (In one study, the researchers successfully trained teachers in mindfulness via telephone instruction!)
- Join a yoga class that centers on meditative or reflective practice. (Yoga that centers on fitness is not likely to develop your mindfulness.)

- Join a class in tai chi or chi gong. Even the classes of some instructors of more vigorous martial arts, like karate, occasionally have a strong focus on mindfulness. If you can't tell from their course materials, ask!
- Join a formal program in Mindfulness-Based Stress Reduction (MBSR). (A great book on MBSR, in fact the original book, is called *Full Catastrophe Living: Using the Wisdom of Your Body and Mind to Face Stress, Pain, and Illness,* by Jon Kabat-Zinn. The book is long and fascinating.)
- Seek out a therapist who specializes in Mindfulness-Based Conceptual Therapy (MBCT).

Gratitude

As a go-getter professional, proud of her strong work ethic, Beth always put success ahead of happiness. Imagine her surprise to learn that not only had she got her priorities exactly backwards, this reversal was driving a good portion of her burnout. Here's her story.

Beth: Getting Happy

In the first pages of Sean Achor's excellent book, *The Happiness Advantage,* the author debunked one of my long-held core beliefs about happiness: *when I succeed, then I'll be happy.* For decades, the notion that success would make me happy had been a cornerstone of my work ethic. Certainly, I do feel great when I achieve something. Sadly, however, that happiness doesn't last.

In fact, Achor says in his book that the *converse* is truer: **When I am happy, then I will succeed.** Was he insisting that success came from creativity and productivity, and that creativity and productivity came much more reliably from happiness than from angst? Yes, in fact, he was. That was news to me!

To build his case, Achor pulled in groundbreaking work by the psychologist Barbara Fredrickson, whose "Broaden and Build" theory has been validated by researchers in a variety of fields. Dr. Fredrickson believes that positive emotions play an essential role in our survival. Other researchers have found that feelings of **love, happiness, joy and gratitude each cause brain function changes that allow for more creative and flexible problem solving.**

Experiencing those positive feelings also give you wider vision, in both literal and figurative senses. *Literal* wider vision: because happiness relaxes your eyes and your nervous system, so that you are able to see not only what's in directly front of you, but also more of what's out to the sides. *Figurative* wider vision, too: in terms of being able to "think outside the box."

In short, when we are happy, it is far easier to face life's inevitable challenges with courage, creativity and vision.

So, how do you support your own happiness? As I said, a terrific first step is to build a habit of gratitude. My inspiring (and super-productive) friend Polly Malby recently wrote to me, *"Enjoy and Make a Difference: I am combining these two goals because I'm realizing that when I infuse joy into everything I do, and am interacting and contributing, I AM making a difference. I am adequate. I don't have to worry. I can still be connected, be authentic, and be A-Okay!"* As Malby so aptly described, this is how growing our happiness can be a key idea for ending burnout and returning to productivity.

Gratitude Builds Happiness

Getting into a habit of expressing gratitude also helps you by bringing your attention to the things you value most in the world. In reviewing the work of gratitude researchers around the world, the Greater Good Project at UC Berkeley is finding that people who practice gratitude consistently report these benefits:

- Stronger immune systems and lower blood pressure
- Higher levels of positive emotions
- More joy, optimism, and happiness
- Acting with more generosity and compassion
- Feeling less lonely and isolated

You'll find some excellent videos on gratitude at the Greater Good project's website: http://greatergood.berkeley.edu/expandinggratitude.

While many people thrive on a daily gratitude practice, others find that their practice becomes rote when they try to do it every single day. Sonja Lyubomirsky, PhD, the researcher-author of another practical book, *The How of Happiness,* suggests that you try writing your gratitude list three times a week, or even once a week. She reports that research shows that for some people, being consistent at this intermittent level of repetition may drive *greater* benefit than an every-day practice of listing the things they are grateful for.

Here is an example of how one person's gratitude list looked. Your own gratitude list may turn out to be more wordy, or much less so.

What Went Well: Susan's Story

Susan Bender Phelps is a good friend of ours. She practices a daily habit of writing about three things that went well each day. Despite a back injury that kept her stuck in bed for nearly two weeks, she did not pause her gratitude practice. Every day she continued to post on her Facebook page about three things that went well. Here is an example from one of her posts during that injury:

"What Went Well: 1. Best day so far for my back. Can get in and out of bed with much more ease. 2. Getting my TSP Executive Board meeting covered as I still can't sit or stand long enough to go in person. 3. Was able to sit and get out some work for a client this morning."

As you can probably guess, Bender Phelps is a vigorous person who makes a habit of accomplishing a great deal. With the two weeks she'd already suffered of flat-on-her-back pain, anyone might excuse her from sticking to her daily "What Went Well" ritual, at least until she felt better. But she was careful not to excuse herself. This exercise was part of her healing process.

We asked her how she got started with her gratitude practice, and why she is so faithful with it. She said she started after a colleague challenged his friends to write a daily gratitude list for just one week. Susan took up the challenge as well and committed fully; that week she wrote her list every day. "I found that I felt so much better, I just kept it going," she told us. "It's become a habit now: I watch my day for things that do go well. It's a wonderful way to pay attention." As of this writing, she has been posting her "three things that went well" for about two years and happily, now that she is feeling much better, she has returned to her busy life as an executive coach, mentor, and public speaker.

Interactive: How Can You Make the Gratitude Habit Work for You?

If you aren't the type to post your gratitude lists on Facebook, you may be like many others who choose to keep their gratitude practices quite private.

There are many ways you can choose to acknowledge and savor the good things in your day. Here are some examples. If you come up with something else that works for you, we'd love to hear about it.

- ☐ Express gratitude to the people around you for the things they do well.
- ☐ If you're having a tough day, remind yourself to find at least one thing you can feel grateful for. (Then, perhaps, one more.)
- ☐ Keep a journal of gratitude lists.
- ☐ Consider holding yourself accountable by regularly posting your gratitude list on social media.
- ☐ Occasionally, read back over some of your lists or posts and allow yourself to savor them again.
- ☐ Institute a family gratitude moment at dinnertime or bedtime. Each person simply lists out loud the good they noticed that day, and what went well.
- ☐ Compose a thank you letter to someone who made a difference in your life. Go into some detail about what you're grateful for, and how it has affected you.
- ☐ If possible, read your thank you letter aloud to its intended recipient. (This is a particularly powerful happiness practice.)
- ☐ Make a collage illustrating things, people and events you are grateful for, and values you treasure. Use personal photographs and mementos, your own artwork or images you clip. Hang the collage where you can see it regularly.

Overcoming Five Pitfalls

Here are five traps for the unwary that can pull people off track with their daily (or weekly) gratitude practices, and simple strategies for staying out of them.

1. Confusing *simple* with *not powerful*. If you are concerned that something as simple as expressing gratitude couldn't possibly be helpful, consider adding, "I enjoy simplicity" to your gratitude practice, and keep on keeping on.
2. Believing that a practice that (at first) may seem hokey or cheesy is also not valuable. Instead, appreciate that this exercise is an antidote to cynicism. (You may remember that is the second of the three dimensions of burnout: Emotional Exhaustion, Cynicism and Inefficacy.)

3. *Neglecting to savor* each item on your gratitude list, as you write or speak it. Take a moment to think about and enjoy, again, each item you are adding to your list.

4. *Forgetting to use habit-building strategies.* Relying on raw will-power uses up your energy, and willpower may thus cease to function when your energy is low. Habit-building strategies include taking a moment to build reminders into your environment (such as scheduling gratitude into your daily calendar, or sticking a one-word note to your dashboard, or posting a photo that reminds you to be grateful). Another strategy is enrolling some supportive partners who will periodically ask you how your gratitude practice is going.

5. *Forgoing variation,* which may allow boredom to sap the value of your gratitude practice. Look at your frequency, style, or audience as ways to change it up. If making a daily list turns out to be too often for you, experiment until you find a recurring routine that works for you. Every other day, three times a week and once a week: all have been shown to have value. Or try playing with a new style of expression to enliven your gratitude practice. You've got so many possibilities: will you choose writing, prayer, drawing or collage, spoken aloud or singing? As for your audience: do you prefer private, or shared? If shared: in person, by phone, on line, by letter or through video?

Celebrate the Small Victories

Recently, we had the honor of leading a Burnout First Aid workshop with a group of public school teachers, administrators, and allied staff. The room was supposed to hold 50 people, but 65 teachers and administrators had joined the workshop.

"What is so routine in your line of work," we asked, "that people long ago stopped acknowledging you for it? In other words, what are the "ordinary" ways that you bring your specialized skills to the kids you work with? How do you facilitate ordinary, everyday miracles, the ones you came into this line of work to see, the ones that feed your heart and soul?"

This question gets at the heart of the third dimension in the burnout triad, fatigue, cynicism and **inefficacy**. Inefficacy is the sense that the work that you do somehow no longer makes a difference. One reason that this occurs is the loss of appreciation and recognition of your everyday use of your professional skills. When you, and other people, cease to appreciate that every day you are superbly executing the fundamental skills of your profession, then it can come to seem like you are hardly doing anything at all. In that atmosphere, it gets very easy to focus only on the problems that you have not yet solved.

You may be feeling like you aren't effective when, in fact, the consistent, skillful, nuanced application of the fundamentals by a knowledgeable professional (like you) is *exactly* what makes a difference! This is why it is so valuable for us to call out and celebrate our everyday small victories. Because those victories are not small. Bit, by bit, by bit, we are building great foundations and changing lives.

What great things do you accomplish, which seem so routine in your line of work that people have stopped acknowledging you for it?

For your inspiration, here is a list of "everyday" accomplishments generated in the workshop by those educational staff, teachers and administrators. Enjoy! What would you include on your own list?

- Use personal, creative ideas to assist students with their own individual needs
- Brief, ongoing communications with special-needs students to facilitate learning motivation
- Customize my training to meet the various needs of my audience
- Thinking & doing "outside the box"
- Creating joy/laughter; Being happy and seeing it become contagious
- Finding & modeling passion
- Playing games
- When a student learns to read or write their first words
- Supporting someone in a difficult situation
- Creating a safe environment for kids who do not have one at home
- Feeding hungry children
- Providing basics: LOVE. Little trinkets!
- Teaching basic skills — such as an orderly way to walk down the hall
- Trying something new
- "Ah-ha" moment, "I get it!"
- Teaching social skills

- Being involved, have the opportunity to have that with staff & students
- Teaching & seeing the results of teaching good manners
- Hiring the right people for our kids (from a principal)
- Empathy — back and forth between students and staff
- Teamwork
- Me time: workouts, windows, coffee
- Meeting a deadline
- Nature!

Interactive: Your "Small" Victories

Consider the questions below and answer with as many examples as possible. Keep the list where you can refer to it and add to it.

For extra benefits (and fun!) get together with a group of people in your profession to create a list together.

What is so seemingly "routine" in your line of work that people may have long ago stopped acknowledging you for it? What are the ordinary ways that you bring your specialized skills to the people and projects you work with? How do you facilitate ordinary, everyday improvements, the ones you came into this line of work to see, the ones that feed your heart and soul?

Identify and Share Your Preferred Recognition Styles

Much has been written about the benefits of recognition — for employees, customers and volunteers — for increasing engagement, motivation and productivity. The business model of many companies is based around building and providing "recognition programs" to other institutions.

But not all people like to be recognized the same way. If you've felt irritated or annoyed by recognition that was given in a "cookie cutter" fashion, or worse, if you've been the focus of recognitions that made you feel painfully uncomfortable, you know that these well-meaning efforts can sometimes increase stress and burnout. If this kind of thing happens to you, let's talk about one reason this may occur and what you can do about it. First, you need just a little background.

In the popular book, *The Five Love Languages,* by Gary Chapman, the author argues that people express love through different styles. By the same token, there are different styles in the ways we wish to receive expressions of love from other people. His five "languages" (many of which are not "said" in words) are:

- Words of affirmation
- Acts of service
- Receiving gifts
- Quality time
- Physical touch

In his book, Chapman says much relationship distress is created by love language mismatches. It can work like this: one person expresses love clearly in their own language style, while the other person is "deaf" to this expression of love, because they don't know enough about the different love languages to even notice their partner's version.

To get past this, Chapman recommends that people in relationships need to take the time to identify their own preferred love language, and learn what their partner's preferred love language is. Can you see how this could dramatically improve each person's experience of the relationship?

Greg Paskal took the concept of "love languages" and modified it for work settings.

Paskal's five **Recognition Styles** are:

- Verbal or Written (actually, for many people, these are two very different styles)

- Acts of service
- Time
- Gifts
- Personal attention

For example, both of us, Dr. Marnie and Beth, love to speak in front of audiences big and small, so public verbal recognition of our accomplishments is a preferred recognition style for both of us. We each would be delighted to be called up in front of large crowd to receive a certificate and say a few words.

However, both of us have friends and family members who detest public recognition. When they are called out in front of an audience, they feel exposed and vulnerable, *even when the callout is entirely positive.* For them, this recognition style feels not like a reward, but a punishment, or at least, a disincentive. The mismatch in delivery style means they are nearly "deaf" to the appreciation. To them, other styles of recognition would feel far more like appreciation.

You'll likely feel some recognition styles warmly support your efforts. At the same time, some might seem token or trivial, some irrelevant, and some might feel downright undesirable.

Take a little time to rank them for yourself, and then share what you've discovered with those who might offer you appreciation. Also, share and discuss the worksheet with those to whom you offer appreciation. For these small efforts, you're likely to garner some big wins for your own morale and motivation, and that of others.

Interactive: Recognition Styles Worksheet
(With appreciation to Greg Paskal and RecognizeAnother.com)

For each recognition style listed below, assign one of these values that best reflects your feelings about that style:

Preferred	Irrelevant
Acceptable	Undesirable
Token	

Verbal (public/private) _____ or
Written (public/private) _____

You appreciate hearing "Good Job," and other affirming words, or getting a card, certificate or other written acknowledgment of a job well done. Indicate if you have a preference for public or private recognition.

Acts of Service _____

You appreciate someone taking the time to help you out or offering assistance. These can be spur of the moment acts; they are usually best when based on the receiver's practical need.

Time _____

You appreciate someone making time for you, even if it's just a few minutes to recognize the effort you have put in. This time is often outside of daily business: coffee, a walk together, lunch.

Gifts _____

You appreciate getting a tangible gift of any value (a small gift is often as effective as a larger one) as a way of saying thank you for something you have done.

Personal Attention _____

You appreciate one-on-one visits with those you are working for, especially when completing difficult or complex tasks. You trust that the visit will not have quality of "looking over your shoulder."

Other _____

You may have other ways you appreciate receiving recognition from others. If so, write them here:

_____

_____

_____

_____

_____

_____

Chapter EIGHT

Capacity: Check the Lay of the Land

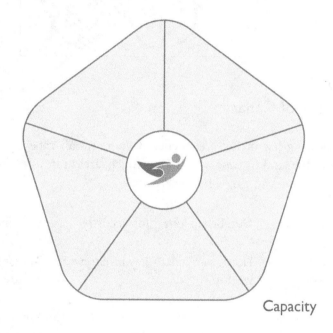

Capacity

"I feel thin, sort of stretched, like butter scraped over too much bread."

—Frodo, *The Fellowship of the Ring*, by J.R.R. Tolkien

Quick check in:

How much do you have on your plate right now? How big was your plate to begin with? What is your maximum capacity for dealing with stress? How close are you to it?

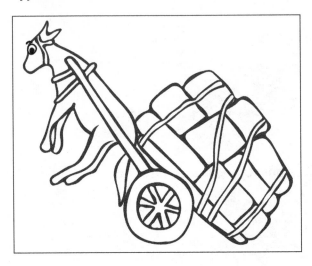

Elements of Capacity

The following list includes elements of your overall capacity. What's the lay of the land in your world? How much stress can you take? How much stress are you currently under?

Job stress level	Number of jobs	Job security	Commute
Standard vs. Shift work	Hours worked/ week	Pay level/reward	Access to nature
On-call	Clear expectations	Level of autonomy	Financial security
Work correspondence	Workload	Sense of fairness	Holmes & Rahe Life Stress Inventory
Responsibilities outside of work	Necessary resources	Alignment of values	Introverted vs Extroverted

As you look through this list, you'll notice a number of these things are simply not within your control. That's okay! Knowing about them is helpful because they have a known impact on your overall stress level. This area can help you prioritize taking action in the parts of your life where you *do* have some sort of control and can therefore have an impact on your overall stress. When it comes to burnout, awareness of your own Capacity and knowing where you can reduce incoming stress is key.

Overall Capacity Goal

Know yourself. Review your Capacity before taking on new responsibilities. If you are quite stressed already, where can you cut back? Recognize that the energy you spend on your work life and home life is coming from just the one you. If you've been feeling stuck or trapped in one area, consider how you might be able to cut stress in another. Since everything is connected through you, any amount of stress relief you can provide yourself can help.

Where to Start

1. **Review** the Capacity elements listed above. (It may be helpful to review your answers from the Capacity Key Area of the Burnout Shield Assessment.)
2. Put a **check mark** by each element of Capacity that you are currently managing well.
3. **Underline** each element of Capacity that you'd like to improve.
4. Of those that you underlined, **circle** any that you are most motivated or feel most equipped to change right now. As you do this, consider whether or not you have the required skills, necessary resources, or control over your schedule, etc.
5. **Rebuild with positive changes.** Fill in the **To Do List** below with your plan for positive changes. *Note: You may want to wait to fill this out until after you've read the rest of the chapter.*

Start where you have indicated you are the most motivated. We recommend that you start with one small change that is easy to incorporate into your daily schedule. Once you've been successful with that positive change, acknowledge your accomplishment and then continue to add more positive changes to your daily routine.

6. **Expand your insight, knowledge and skill level:** As you read on, you'll learn more about the different elements of Capacity and how they impact your health and your ability to withstand burnout. We share some of our own stories and stories from the people that we've helped. You'll also find some additional resources and assessment tools that can help you become more familiar with aspects of Capacity.

Considering how vast these topics are, this chapter is intended only as a guide to some elements of Capacity that are most directly related to your ability to withstand burnout.

However, we encourage you to reach beyond this book. There are so many helpful Capacity resources out there, and they can be the doorway to a great deal of healing of your strength.

Capacity To-Do List

Positive change under my control that I will try first:

_____

_____

_____

Positive changes I am interested to try in the near future:

_____

_____

_____

Positive changes I may incorporate someday, but will put aside until I've successfully incorporated the changes listed above:

_____

_____

_____

Capacity Results

Positive changes that have made the greatest difference in my life:

_____

_____

_____

Elements of Capacity that I tend to let slip when I am under stress:

_____

_____

_____

Helpful Capacity reminder for myself the next time I'm under stress:

_____

_____

_____

Positive Changes

Here are some examples of positive changes you can make for the different elements of Capacity:

Job Stress Level; Standard vs. Shift Work, On-Call; Work Correspondence
- These areas tend to be outside of your control, but recognize these factors as potential sources of stress.

- Connect with resources, support groups for people in similar stressful circumstances.

Responsibilities Outside of Work
- Keep one calendar that allows you to track work and personal events.
- Identify activities that benefit you in one of the other Burnout Shield areas — keep these in your schedule.
- Identify activities that do not benefit you in one of the other Burnout Shield areas — delay, delegate or drop these.

Number of Jobs; Hours worked/week
- Look for one job that would pay you enough to allow you to drop one of the other ones.
- If hourly, be sure your workplace is following legal standards for tracking all hours worked, overtime, breaks, etc.
- If salary or self-employed, prioritize your time for work that is important and urgent. Leave unimportant, non-urgent work for a later time.

Clear expectations; Workload
- Clarify expectations with supervisors. If verbal, send an email to confirm you understood all the points.
- Keep a visible list of current projects (in order of priority) and new assignments.
- Seek technology or training that may help you do your work more efficiently.

Necessary resources
- Clearly communicate your need for any additional resources.
- Check with others who do your type of work; can you collaborate or share?
- Seek creative ways to obtain the resources you need.

Job security; Pay level/reward
- Have a backup plan and keep your resume current.
- Ask for a raise. Be the squeaky wheel. It is unlikely to happen if you never ask!

- Adjust your expectations. Recognize the non-financial benefits of working at your current job.

Level of autonomy; Sense of fairness; Alignment of values
- Seek opportunities which will allow you greater control over your work.
- Bring any perceived unfairness to the attention of your supervisor. Show how it lowers productivity.
- Clarify your organization's mission and values. If they are not in line with yours, identify ways in which working at this job fits within your stated values.

Commute; Access to nature
- Find ways to reduce the stress of your commute: travel at non-peak times, ride share, listen to relaxing music or books on tape, walk or bike.
- Change your commute to a more scenic route.
- Put a plant (or an image of a nature scene) within view of your workstation.

Financial security
- Track your spending.
- Take advantage of one of the many debt management resources available.
- Watch the documentary *I'm Fine, Thanks,* about resetting financial expectations.

Holmes & Rahe Life Stress Inventory
- Since the events measured on this scale happened in the past, they are outside of your control.
- Use this scale to help you identify the impact that current stressful events may have.

Introverted vs extroverted
- Align the expectations you have for yourself with the reality of who you are.
- If you are more introverted, prioritize time alone to recharge your energy.

- If you are more extroverted, prioritize time with others to recharge your energy.

In Simple Terms: Your Bucket

A simple analogy for thinking about your stress capacity is thinking of water in a bucket. A bucket can only hold so much water. If your bucket is fairly empty, a drop or two won't make much of a difference, but if your bucket is filled to the brim, a drop or two can cause a spill.

Your stress capacity is the same way. If you aren't under much stress at the time, an activity here or an emotionally demanding situation there won't make much of a difference, but if your "bucket" is already full, it won't take much more to put you over the edge.

So what can be done about this bucket of yours? You can either increase the size of your bucket (which not be possible) or you can get rid of some of the water you are carrying.

Let's consider that "water," otherwise known as stress. It's time to look at all the sources of stress in your life and exert control in the areas where you can. Brace yourself — this may mean breaking commitments, changing plans, and delegating or delaying projects. If you find yourself resistant to this thought, think: what will happen if your burnout becomes so debilitating that you can't honor your commitments anyway? It is better to lighten your load in an orderly fashion.

You may be surprised at how easy much of this process can be. If you are burned out, the people around you are probably very aware of this. At the minimum, they won't be surprised that you need to lighten your load, and at the most, they will be happy to help. Of course, try to steer away from handing things off to someone else who is also burned out.

A Common Obstacle

Be prepared for a surprising, yet common, obstacle: you. Some of the hardest things to unload from your stress bucket are the things you put there yourself. These are the things that you took on because you thought they were important. Nobody asked you, though you may now feel accountable for them since you've declared that you would be.

If you've experienced any sort of hardship in order to continue your commitment to this goal, it is going to be even harder to give it up. The psychological process that leads to such commitment is the same that makes hazing so powerful. It is hard to admit that we've purposefully done something to cause ourselves harm. So when we are faced with evidence that we've willingly put ourselves in harm's way, we often tell ourselves that there must be a very good reason for it. We start to assign an even bigger value to that initial goal. "I allowed myself to be hurt, this thing must *really* be worth it. Otherwise, what the heck is wrong with me? I'm not stupid. No. So it must be super important." But is it? The longer this process continues and the greater the harm we allow ourselves to endure, the stronger this inflated sense of value, and the resulting bond to the goal, can get.

Marnie: Sometimes It's Best to Let It Go

I once counseled a student who was dealing with this kind of issue, and we came up with a fun way to help her remember that it wasn't worth the cost of sticking with it. Here's a bit of her back-story: she had a lot going on in her life. Her Holmes and Rahe Life Stress Inventory score was incredibly high, and her many work and school commitments were pushing her to her limit. In addition to all of this, one of her major sources of stress was a personal matter that she spent a great deal of time and energy trying to fix.

Someone she cared about was in a relationship where she was afraid that person might get hurt. However, as we discussed it more, it became evident that the people in this situation were consenting adults. Nothing illegal was happening, it wasn't an issue that affected her directly, it wasn't even a situation where she had been asked to help; in fact, her help wasn't even desired. She was doing this because she really wanted to protect a person she cared about from potential harm. Her intentions were admirable, but in the end, her efforts were a bit of a lost cause.

This all happened at a time when the movie *X Men: First Class* had been recently released. I compared her situation to the scene where a young Magneto is desperately trying to hold on to the submarine of his nemesis as it dove deeper and deeper under the water. Magneto was in a situation that meant very much to him, but if he continued with it in the same way, it would destroy him. As we talked more, my student realized that this situation with her loved one was her "submarine" and she was being pulled deeper and deeper under water. She had done as much as she could. If she continued to hold on, spending time or energy on this issue, it had the real potential to break her, or at the least, cause her to fail classes and be kicked out of school. So she decided to drop the issue.

I remember how relieved she seemed when she realized that she could really be done with the matter. To remind her of this, I printed out a screenshot of Magneto holding onto the submarine and asked her to look at it if she ever found herself thinking she had to intervene in that relationship again. She laughed when I handed it to her, but months later, she returned to my office and told me that she would look back at that picture whenever she needed a reminder to stay focused on the things that mattered the most to her right now.

Strategies for Improving Your Capacity

Here, we're offering six strategies for improving your capacity:

- Schedule a self-check
- Recognize the value of what you are already doing
- Say no
- Delay, delegate and drop
- Make time for fun
- Align with your inner nature

Schedule a Self-Check

Doing a self-check includes a second step that ensures you continue the habit:

- Do the self-check
- Immediately schedule another self-check

When you answered the Capacity Key Area of the Burnout Shield Self-Tests, were you already fully aware that you have been attempting to carry an almost-impossible load of responsibilities and stresses? Or were you startled (as many are) by the unreasonably heavy load you've accumulated?

Either way, it helps to begin this process by becoming aware of your actual current stress load. This step is required in order to pare your load back to something you'd reasonably expect to be able to carry, or to keep you from going over your limit if you aren't yet there.

Take inventory: **What's on your plate? What is *everything* on your plate? Is this a reasonable load? Give yourself credit!**

Doing a periodic re-assessment of your stress load is also key to keeping your Capacity where you need it to be. Many responsible and dedicated people tend to add tasks and responsibilities without ever removing any. You can guard against this dangerous tendency by opening your calendar *right now* and scheduling another Capacity self-check. Start by putting the next one in the calendar at a date three months from now. You'll learn as you go what the best time interval for you will be.

Recognize the Value of What You Are Already Doing

As burnout makes itself felt, many of us may come to feel that our efforts are less and less valuable. Feeling that you can no longer make a difference is a classic dimension of burnout itself, one of the "big three:" exhaustion, cynicism and a **low sense of personal accomplishment**. Please remember that it isn't that you are actually ineffective, just that you *feel* ineffective.

In order to help yourself out of burnout, you'll need to see past this illusion. Two main ways to do this are by reflecting and by gaining an outside perspective. As discussed in Chapter 7, daily reflection on your personal values, with an honest assessment of how those values were supported during the events of the day, can help you recover your sense of purpose. As discussed in Chapter 9, getting perspective from someone you trust, such as a mentor or a counselor, can help you to gain an objective view of your value and effectiveness.

Notice the Ripples You Create

Sometimes it takes a while before you learn the value of your efforts. Your work and the effect you have on others can create ripples that spread outward from yourself. It may be a long time before you learn what other shore they reach or how they've affected others. When you get this type of feedback from others, we recommend you keep track of it! When someone says, "What you did made a difference," or, "What you did meant so much to me that I am now paying it forward," it indicates how much value you have to others.

- Tip: Keep a "kudos file" of any notes of praise or thanks that you receive from others.

Marnie: Keep a Kudos File

When I first went into practice, my father recommend that I start a "kudos" file, where I could keep track of my patient thank-you notes (along with a copy in their charts, of course). He said it wouldn't be something I'd look at often, but it was a good idea to have in any high-stakes position. "Looking back on the words of people you've helped is the best way to get through any tough times you might have ahead." Boy, was he right! On the days when I was feeling especially defeated, I'd take an extra 30 seconds in my office and gently glance through the file. Those notes and cards were incredible medicine. They helped me reenergize and feel ready to greet my next patient with a full heart and a renewed sense of optimism.

Beth: Those Ripples May Reach a Farther Shore

At first, I focused solely on worrying about the people whom it seemed I could not help, (such as the pregnant teenager who persisted eating a diet of junk food, despite all my efforts to help her see the need to better support her baby's growth and her own.) Yet, while I was focusing on what I *couldn't* do, I was overlooking all that I *had been* doing. Looking back, I see that I was also receiving messages that my efforts were generating benefits I could not see. For example: a year after she graduated, one of my former students came back to thank me for being (in her mind) "present at her side" at all of the first one hundred births she had attended in her first job of her career.

Strategies for Decreasing Your Stress

Evaluate Your Work Situation

One of the upsides of saving yourself from burnout is that you get the perfect opportunity to step back and look at some of life's "big picture" issues. In this case, how well is your current work situation working for you? Keep in mind that you might be feeling ineffective at work, and feeling that way could actually be a symptom of your burnout, not a reflection of reality.

However, before you were feeling burned out, were you feeling well matched with your current job? Is your skill set well suited for the type of work you are doing? Are you working for an organization that treats you fairly? Does it align with your values? Is there possibly a different occupation that you'd enjoy more? This might be the time to reevaluate your career choices to see if there is a better match for you out there.

Books such as *What Color is Your Parachute* by Richard Nelson Bolles, and *StrengthsFinder 2.0* by Tom Rath can be useful in helping you to evaluate whether or not your skills and personality attributes are well matched for your current position. Even if you don't feel it is possible to change careers at this point, it may be helpful to use these or other tools to identify what your strengths are so that you can go about utilizing them in your current position as much as possible.

How about your current work schedule? Is there a way to change your hours to better suit your personal needs? If you are working a swing shift, is it possible to switch to a more standard work schedule? If your workday never seems to end, can you establish times that you will and will not be available to answer after-hours work correspondence? If you are encountering long delays in traffic during your daily commute, is it possible to shift the start and end time of your workday? Just starting an hour earlier and leaving an hour later can help you avoid those high-traffic times.

As you go through this process, please consider having a counselor, mentor or other objective third party review these issues with you. You may have been coping with certain issues for so long that you may not realize how unusual they were in the first place, or perhaps you've forgotten that they can actually change! An outside perspective can be especially useful during this process.

Say No

In this chapter, we are looking at your capacity to take on stress and your current stress load. It is important that you know your limits and know how close you are to them.

Why is it so important that you learn to say no more often? Because if you are precariously close to your limits, or are over your stress limits, it is important that you say no to new sources of stress and start getting some of the existing sources of stress off your plate.

If you are experiencing burnout, the chances are good that you, like us, tend to take on a lot. Check in with yourself. Were you raised with a notion of "it is better to give than to receive?" Of course doing nice things for others adds meaning and pleasure to life. But even if you are only giving gifts of your energy and time, it isn't always sustainable to give and give. Have you conditioned yourself to say "yes" to everything without realizing why?

As health care providers, our patients' needs always come first. Maybe for you, it's your students' needs, your children's needs, or your clients' needs. The needs of the people we serve can seem so much more visible and important than our own. However, if you allow yourself to break, how will you possibly continue to help them? Your needs are a priority as well.

It is time to ask yourself: have you taken the virtues of generosity and caring way past your human limits? Beth did — here is her story:

Beth: Exceeding My Limits

Here's what happened to me when I gave and gave and gave until I exceeded my own human limits.

For years, I gave everything I had. I accepted the extra shifts, the committee work and the volunteer work. I skimped on sleep. I answered the phone. I dragged my body out the door.

My clients loved me, and I lived to serve. It was my joy and my calling. But eventually, to continue to get it all done, I found I wasn't just "borrowing" from tomorrow's energy. I felt like I was using up my *next year's* energy.

Sadly, my own children remember me in those years as sometimes a "mom-zombie." Because I poured so much of my energy into my patients, caring for my children (the children who had the keys to my heart!) ceased, at times, to be my joy. I did not feel good about this, but I did not really understand burnout, then.

Eventually, the zombie-me ended up going through the motions at work, too. Work was no longer my joy, either.

All that time, I had been ignoring my body's various signals about its limits. My personal "Achilles' heel" is chronic asthma. I knew perfectly well that, like other autoimmune illnesses, asthma is made worse by stress and poor diet. But, as with many people with burnout, I simply ignored my physical warning signs and carried on.

Finally, my health fell apart in a way I could not ignore. That day, I was driving to a hair salon I had visited many times before. During the trip, I suddenly became frightened because I could not figure out where I was.

Later, I came to realize that my poor body suddenly had no more reserves. I had been ignoring all my asthma symptoms, using my rescue inhaler more and more and more as I kept on going at my usual pace. My brain had slowly become so oxygen-starved from asthma that this day, I couldn't even recognize familiar landmarks.

I called my husband. He rushed out of work to bring me to an Emergency Room. The ER doctor admitted me to the hospital, and for the next few days they pumped me full of medications with remarkably unpleasant side effects.

Thus began my *year* on full disability from work, while I slowly recovered my health. Did that experience mean I had learned my lesson? Well, no, not really. Not enough. I am sorry to say that when I finally was able to go back to work, I was only slightly more cautious about over-giving. It took several more years before I finally learned about burnout and how I kept falling into it.

As I now understand it, burnout's relationship to those who are over-giving is twofold:

1. Giving is great. Making the world a better place is really great. Offering your deeply-knowledgeable skills is a wonderful thing.

However:
2. If you consistently and routinely push past your human limits, then burnout *will* set in.

Burnout means you lose your enthusiasm and your ability to care. You may even trash your health, like I did. Once that happens, it can be a long, long road back. Here's the question I should have asked myself then; I offer it now to you. I hope it arrives in time to prevent your (next) falling-apart moment:

If you don't respect your own limits, then how will you continue to serve your clients, your students or your family?

Ways to Say NO

Make Them Wait
If you're thinking of saying *yes:* Build in a pause — at least 24 hours — before you answer. "Thanks for asking! I need to think about it. I'll I get back to you by _____" is a great answer. Then

do think about it. Try making a pros and cons list. Ask a trusted colleague or friend for their input.

Train Them to Expect Delayed Responses

Do you find that your time is never your own? Are you plagued by a lack of time to focus deeply on your own projects? Consider training your clients or constituents to expect a delayed response from you when they make requests.

Find ways to structure an environment where this is expected. For instance, this might include changing your voicemail message to incorporate a phrase like, "My office hours are from 10–6," or, "I return calls right after lunch and from 4–5 pm each weekday," or, even, "I return calls on the next business day."

Here is another great example of training your correspondents to expect delayed responses. It comes from Kim, the leader of a busy high-end web design company.

Kim prides herself on providing super-responsive customer service and instant responses to her employees' questions. However, this level of service has also generated constant interruptions for her busy production schedule. She felt an increasingly desperate need to claw back some of her time from the constant interruptions.

A few months ago, despite her fear that her clients and employees might resent her lack of availability and her business might suffer as a result, she set up this autoresponder message in her business email:

"Happy Friday, and thanks for contacting me! This is an *automated message* to let you know that today is a deep focus day here at our office. We're minimizing email to create space for intense brainstorming, super-charged coding, and completing challenging client projects. If your email is received before noon, you will get an answer by the end of the day. Otherwise, we look forward to answering your question on Monday."

(To make sure she got full value from this strategy, Kim also trained herself not to open any work emails after noon on Friday.)

To Kim's astonishment, her clients and employees *love* this email! They tell her that reading it gives them pleasure, and also leads them to admire Kim's work ethic even more. Perhaps because she coupled the act of carving out her own time with a clear explanation of its value to her constituents, this tactic of pushing them away on Friday afternoons has won increased respect from the very people she is training to wait for her response.

Interactive: Train Them to Wait

Whom do you need to teach to expect delayed responses, and how will you consistently train them to expect delays?

_____

_____

_____

Anticipate and Calendar

A great reason to say no is because you already have "prior commitments." So create some that serve you.

Every three to six months, perhaps during your self-check, sit down with your calendar and block out time for important personal events. For example: the weekend of your cousin's wedding, your kids' soccer games, and your vacation days. While you're at it, commit yourself to some quiet evenings at home, as well. Then make sure to put in for the time off your work schedule, too, if that's required. Are you one of the millions who don't use all their vacation days every year? Schedule those days! The breaks will improve your overall health and productivity.

Next, proceed to fiercely protect all these commitments. Say, "I'm so sorry, I have a prior commitment on Wednesday evenings." It's up to you whether you share with them that your standing Wednesday appointment is game night with the family or a Zumba class. These activities are important because they protect you from burnout. They deserve to be in your schedule. They deserve your time.

Don't Brood, Act

Is there someone in your life who continually disrespects your time boundaries? It is a common response to wait for days or weeks for a "good time" to speak up. However, if someone tramples on your time boundaries, don't brood over it. Sitting on your concerns for days or weeks before you speak up allows these behaviors to continue unchecked.

The most powerful time to speak up is right at the moment the transgression occurs. Practice these sentences below so that when one of your lines has been crossed, you can handle it in an immediate and effective manner.

Be Specific

As you speak up, avoid vague explanations like "I'm too stressed." Put your explanation in terms that support your boss' or your organization's goals. "I'm currently working on a high priority project. If you want me to work on this, I'll be able to start it on ＿＿＿＿＿＿." or "I'm already at my workload capacity right now. We've been instructed to reduce liability by keeping our patients/customers safe, and also keeping their patient satisfaction scores high."

If your supervisor is the one who constantly pushes you past your boundaries, seek their input in prioritizing your work list and identifying what can be delayed or dropped entirely.

Document

If documentation will help support you in defending the limits you've set, track the time you spend on each project. Either on paper, or using one of the many apps that are now available, **record** the time you spend on each project or client. For instance, you might use this record to help you present data that shows all of the valuable things you are already doing.

How to Say No—Phrases to Practice

Practice! Get yourself to the point where you can say these phrases without hesitation. Remember, this isn't personal. This is a statement of fact. The bucket is full. A limit is a limit. Say these phrases with confidence and pride in your value.

- That project deserves attention but unfortunately, I'm not available.
- No, I'm not available to help you with that right now. (If there is a future time when you will be available, tell them. If not, refer them to another resource if available.)
- No, that's not going to work. (Give an alternate solution if available.)
- I have a prior commitment.

- My schedule is currently full. That's not something I can participate in (at this time.)
- I would like to give this the attention and energy it deserves. So that I can do that, which of my current priorities would you like me to drop?

Delay, Delegate and Drop

Once you've reviewed the full spread of commitments you are already carrying, recover your Capacity by mastering the Three D's: Delay, Delegate and Drop.

Delay. *What can you postpone?* Are you able to put some commitments off until a time when you will genuinely be less busy? The pitfall here can be that your perception of your future self may be distorted. Your actual future may not feel emotionally real to you. Brain scans have shown that some people's view of their future self actually exists in a different part of their brain than their present self. Their future self lives in a part of the brain reserved for models of other people, not themselves.

If this is true for you, then while your present self is overwhelmed, your future self exists in an ideal cognitive space where problems and challenges are far less real. If this is the case, it can be easy to assign work to your less-real future self.

There's a simple way to resolve this problem so that your future self becomes real to you and you can reasonably assign yourself future tasks and goals. Further research has shown that practicing positive meditation about your ideal future self can help end the sense of conceiving of your future self as a different person.

Delegate. *Who else could or should be doing this?* Can you allow it to be done differently than you would do it? A great book to read on this topic is the classic *The One Minute Manager Meets the Monkey,* by Kenneth Blanchard, William Oncken and Hal Burrows. You don't have to carry the job title of "manager" to get a lot of value from this little book.

Drop. *Lighten the load.* Start by making this guideline for yourself: *when you add a new commitment, a current commitment has to go.* Here is how you might make this point to your boss: "What project would you like me to defer or drop from my current list so that this new task can get the attention it needs?"

A subcategory of **Drop**: use the two-list principle to mercilessly (and productively) **pare your priority list**. If applicable (or necessary), include your boss in this process. The strategy goes like this:

1. **Make a list of your top 25** projects and priorities.
2. **Identify your top 5 projects and priorities. Do this by crossing out secondary priorities** on that list, until you're left with just 5. (If you are having trouble deciding because they are *all* important, try walking down your list as a set of pairs, like this: Is 1 or 2 more important to me? Cross out the lesser of those two, and compare the winner with #3. Cross out the lesser in that pair, and compare the winner with #4. And so on.)
3. **Discipline yourself to *ignore* your other 20 priorities** and projects until you've accomplished your top 5.

Make Time for Fun

"Fun? Leisure? Are you kidding me? I have too much to do!"

"I don't even remember what I used to do for fun. I wish I did. I feel guilty even thinking about it."

Sound familiar?

How Guilt & Wishful Thinking Can Kill Fun and Increase Burnout

Are you feeling some resistance to the very idea that you need to take some time out for fun? You are not alone. Guilt and wishful thinking can kill fun and increase burnout. Yet many professions have a big population of people who feel guilty about taking time out. Naming just a few:

- Academics and schoolteachers
- Medical students, residents and doctors
- Attorneys
- Clergy
- Social workers and psychotherapists
- Parents

Dreaming of a Break? Do It!

When we finally do realize we need a break, many of us try to cope with this need by wishful thinking. Do you see pictures of other people on vacation and wish that could be you? Or do you yearn after a chance to hike in the woods? If all you are doing is wishing but you never plan anything, this may feel like harmless daydreaming, a mental vacation, or even "thinking positively," but as Gabriele Oettingen points out in her research-based book, *Rethinking Positive Thinking: The New Science of Motivation*, this oft-recommended strategy of daydreaming can actually get in your way. You can't meet your need successfully by this emotion-focused coping technique.

For example, for professionals in the ministry, "while leisure behavior and leisure satisfaction helped decrease burnout, leisure attitude had no effect." In other words, getting out there and doing something fun was great for reducing clergy burnout. It didn't matter if the clergy person felt guilty, or believed leisure was an important use of their time. It just mattered if they actually *did something*, for fun, outside of work.

Try Thanking Yourself

Please don't kick yourself if you find you've been indulging in wishful thinking. If you're emotionally exhausted (a prime component of burnout), it is likely that you have been resisting change, even positive change, in order to "protect your remaining resources." Your wishful thinking could be a result of that protective instinct. This is only natural. However, watch out for protective instincts that go on for too long and become part of the overall problem. If you are then feeling guilty about the resistance, that feeling will also add to the stress.

As you know if you've tried, it's almost impossible to ignore guilt, or "just let it go." Instead, try to bring curiosity and gratitude to these difficult feelings. It might sound something like this inside your own head: "Oh, guilt and wishful thinking, here you are again! That must mean I am wanting to protect my energy and my resources. What touched that off for me?...You are so right; I do need to take care of myself here. Thank you for bringing that to my attention. Now, let me see, what is a better way I could steward my energy today?" This moves us from guilt and wishing, through curiosity, to gratitude, while avoiding self-criticism.

This self-talk may sound a little silly or sappy at first. You're certainly welcome to re-frame your curiosity and gratitude in any way that works for you. But the research is clear: even the American College of

Surgeons is recommending people cultivate gratitude to avoid burnout. Why not apply some of that gratitude to yourself?

Now that we've moved the guilt about leisure a little aside, let's take a look at how leisure activities impact burnout.

Socialize and Move the Body

Medical students definitely have extremely busy lives. Nevertheless, having personal lives that include leisure activities has been shown to reduce their stress and improve their resilience. On the flip side, medical students who engaged in "inadequate social activity" were noted to have decreased mental health. (In that same study, the researchers even noted that wishful thinking had a bad effect on medical students' life satisfaction.)

As you may expect, exercise frequently shows up as a prime mover in the department of feel better and decrease burnout. We are certainly fans of moving the body, because movement can counter inertia, sluggishness, and brain fog.

However, the following words of caution may be especially needed for those of you who are burned out and still pushing yourselves to keep on keeping on. (You know who you are!)

If your burnout has progressed to physical exhaustion or illness, be gentle with yourself. If you are ill or seriously exhausted, your first priorities need to be: get help, get well and get at least somewhat rested before you engage in rigorous exercise!

Music, Games, Fun

"I don't even remember what I used to do for fun!" Did this sentence resonate for you? If so, it's likely that you're deep in burnout. The two first dimensions of burnout, emotional exhaustion and cynicism (or callousness or numbness) may have you in their grip.

Try participating in music or games. In a post on the wonderful website GreaterGood.com, Jill Suttie lists four great ways that music strengthens social bonds:

1. Music increases contact, coordination, and cooperation with others
2. Music gives us an oxytocin boost (oxytocin is the bonding and trust hormone)

3. Music strengthens our "theory of mind" and empathy. Music makes us better at understanding other people
4. Music increases cultural cohesion

Lynda Sharpe, in a long but fun article published by *Scientific American* in May 2011, reviewed the evidence for resilience and stress reduction. She concluded that the most important benefits of children's play may not be (as previously thought) practicing adult skills. In fact, she says the most important function of play — at any age — may well be stress reduction and resilience.

Enjoying yourself in ways you choose for yourself (because you love them) helps to increase life satisfaction, and decreases burnout. Furthermore, after you take a break, you'll often find leisure has improved your engagement. Go ahead and thank your guilty feelings and wishful thinking, because they are natural and informative. And then replace them with play-in-action.

When is it Time to Eat the Marshmallow?

Have you heard of the Stanford Marshmallow experiments? These famous experiments on willpower were originally done in the 1960's. They tested small children, ages 4 to 6, to find out which ones had the self-control to resist eating a marshmallow for 15 minutes. They'd leave the child alone in a room, with the instruction, "You can eat that one marshmallow on the plate right now, if you want. OR you can have TWO marshmallows if you wait to eat them until I come back." Then they'd observe each child through a one-way mirror. Some kids found ways to resist the siren call of that one marshmallow for the whole 15 minutes. Some broke down and ate it before the researcher re-entered the room.

They then followed these children for decades. As they grew older, the children who had had the willpower to "delay gratification," (in other words, willfully delay their pleasure) and not eat the marshmallow right away, tended to have far better outcomes in their lives. They tended to have higher SAT scores, higher graduation rates, higher income, and so on and so forth. The researchers reasoned that this illustrated how important willpower is, and how much impact it can have on future outcomes in that person's life.

There's some scientific disagreement about what the marshmallow experiments actually proved about those kids. Perhaps some of them were better at following directions from authorities? But most agree that it measured the ability to be self-disciplined and delay gratification.

Here's our point: for those of you dealing with burnout, is it possible that you have become *too* good at deferring your gratification, at putting off your pleasure? While there's no question that this skill has enabled you to accomplish a great deal in your lives, is it possible that you've gotten to the point where you've cut out too much pleasure? Whatever your personal "marshmallows" may be, have you gone from delaying gratification to *denying* gratification?

You know what they say about "all work and no play:" it makes Jack a dull boy. And it makes Jill a dull girl, too. Perhaps all this time, that saying has been a statement on burnout. By *dull*, they meant brain fog and low productivity. Burnout.

Interactive: Is It Time to Eat the Marshmallow?

What pleasures and gratifications have you been denying yourself? Which of life's "marshmallows" have you almost never let yourself get around to eating? Write them here:

_____

_____

_____

_____

_____

_____

_____

Ideas for Leisure Activities from Fellow Burnout-Fighters

If you're someone who has trouble prioritizing leisure activities, it may be time for you to recognize their value in helping you successfully resist burnout. Perhaps one or two of these ideas (some of which are pretty quirky) from our friends and advisees will catch your interest, or spark an idea for your own life "marshmallow" — or even s'more — that's not on this list.

Here are some of our favorite examples of things people do for a break or fun.

- 20 minutes of sitting silently and alone, just breathing, every day at lunchtime. Crystal, the dental hygienist who told me about this, said that when she doesn't make this time, the afternoon in their very busy office gets much harder for her to manage.

- Blue sky break. Kristin, the school social worker who shared this, said that her office had a window that showed a small patch of blue sky. It was the only blue sky (or clouds!) that she saw during her working day, so she would look up and just let her mind and heart sail into the sky for just a few moments between crises.

- Stretch breaks. Kim, the extremely analytical and task-oriented programmer who shared this with us, said that, the way she operates, she HAS to do everything on her to-do list. So these days, she makes sure that a 20-minute walk and a 20-minute stretch break are listed on her to-do list every day.

- Play with a pet. If you have a pet, incorporate time with them into your schedule. Throw a ball for a dog for 10 minutes. Dangle a string for your cat. Read aloud to your guinea pig — who will love it! (Really and truly. Karen, a hardworking adult, eventually read aloud a couple of the books from the Game of Thrones series to her guinea pig, a few ages at a time. "He loved it!" she said. "I just had to read every page in my most cheerful voice, and he was delighted. He clearly thought each chapter was about everyone enjoying delicious carrots together.")

- Scheduled monthly massages. Susan bought a year's subscription for monthly massages from a spa she likes. Those appointments are not gifts for other people, they go on *her* to-do list. For Susan, paying for them ahead of time is key, because she wouldn't dream of wasting the money by not going for the massages.

- Forest hikes. Devorah lives near a big city park that is densely forested. She makes it a point to get out for a walk in the forest at least several times a week. "That's my happy place," she says.

- Role playing games. Role-playing games (RPGs) are played by groups of people in which each person assumes the role of a character in a fictional world. There are no winners or losers, and the players tend to work together as a group to solve problems or accomplish goals. Dungeons and Dragons was one of the first, but now there are dozens of games in at least as many different genres. Visit a gaming store to find out what types of gamers meet in your area. Our friend Mario, a Navy vet turned high-powered salesman, swears by get-togethers for table-top role play for reducing his stress.

- Watercolor painting. A couple of years ago, Syrena, a department manager at an extremely busy and fast-growing corporation, began posting her attempts at watercolor paintings to her Facebook page. "This is just for fun," she would post. "I think I'm getting just a little better at painting water." Or trees. Or faces. Of course, her paintings were novice-level, for the first year or so. But we were so impressed that she kept doing it. It was obviously fun for her. Two years later, her paintings are getting pretty good! Occasionally, she takes classes and goes to museum events. But mostly she just paints. For fun. Another version of this: another friend, Janice, got fascinated by body painting, and takes many classes in this art form.

- Paint miniatures or models. You can buy the models — and the paints — at craft stores and also at table-top gaming stores.

- Design and sew costumes.

- Cosplay. 'Costumed Play.' Our friend Damien loves dressing up and pretending to be a fictional character (usually a sci-fi, comic book, or anime character.) If this sounds like fun for you, you can even find whole conferences for people who meet to share their cosplay.

- Quilting.

- Keep an art journal. Your journal is a private place where you paint, draw, create collages or scrapbook.

- Attend an improvisational theater class. Many of our friends have gone to improv class to loosen up, find more humor in life, and become more responsive to others. (Our friend Tara Rolstad, founder of Shattering Stigma and co-author of the book, *No, Really, We WANT You to Laugh*, did this. Tara eventually turned her incredibly stressful life experiences into her life's work — by learning to transform her own tragic and difficult life experiences into hilariously funny comedy bits. Now she helps others learn to do the same.)

- Choir. For one year, Beth sang in a community choir with an amazing director. "I loved the music, which was at a complexity that was quite challenging for me. For the 90 minutes of practice, I did not — could not! — think about one thing except the beautiful music."

- Social club. We both adore our Toastmasters Club. The members are definitely our "tribe." We laugh and learn and grow with them. Kristi feels this way about her Rotary Club. By the way, in any membership group — from Rotary to BNI to church clubs — the personalities of the members and culture of each chapter can vary widely. If you want to try out a social organization, visit different local chapters until you find one with members and culture that are fun and welcoming for *you*.

Align With Your Inner Nature

How well do you fit with your workplace culture and the nature of your work? The shape of your "bucket" (how much stress you can handle) depends in part on aspects of your personality and temperament. These aspects may also make you more susceptible to burnout, depending on how well you know yourself and how well you navigate through or around situations that might be especially tough for you.

Because they are hard-wired elements of your personality, difficult or even impossible to change, they affect the way you deal with stress. The big lesson here is to know yourself as well as possible, to know which situations might create more stress than others and to accommodate your own individual needs. Make sure you are well matched with the challenges you face.

Let's use the analogy of a vehicle. If you are driving a vehicle and have to drive under bridges or choose parking spots, you really need to know the dimensions of the vehicle you are driving, right? Are you in a compact car, an SUV or a big box truck? Some are better suited for going under bridges and fitting in tight parking spaces than others.

People are the same way, but about the type of stress they can handle and how they handle it.

As the author Anais Nin wrote, "We don't see things as they are, we see things as we are." It is natural to assume that everyone thinks and feels the same way you do and that everyone would react the same way in a given situation. This is why it is so important to be aware of your own tendencies and biases; that way you aren't blind to the way they affect your reactions and decisions.

Here are some aspects to consider:

- **Are you an extrovert or an introvert?** If you tend to feel energized by participating in group activities or interacting with a crowd of people, you are likely an extrovert. If these activities overstimulate you and you'd prefer activities where you get to think deeply, reflect and focus on one thing, you are likely an introvert. It isn't necessarily an all-or-nothing thing, but if you have a tendency to be one way over the other, it can help to know which types of activities will help to re-energize you throughout your day. It is also worth noting that while studies have shown introverts have a higher susceptibility to burnout, either type can develop it.

- **Are your core values in line with your organization?** Are you doing work that is meaningful to you? Is the company you work for one that shares any of your core values? A mismatch between your values and the values of the place you work can create a great deal of stress. In fact, this is one of the six main areas of "mismatch," identified by researchers Christine Maslach. PhD and Michael Leiter, PhD, that are most likely to lead to burnout.

  If you need help identifying your core values, there are many books and online tools to help you do so. If you are bothered by a mismatch in this area, it may help to explore more about the nature of the company you work for and the way their work affects the community. Perhaps there is more meaning to the work than you know. If not, and if this is an area that causes you a great deal of stress, it is important to acknowledge that. It may mean that it is time to find work that is more meaningful to you, or at least participate in activities after work that are meaningful to you.

  On the other hand, if you know your work isn't meaningful to you, but you continue to work there because it is a way to make money, that's significant as well. In that case, focus on the meaningful things in your private life that your employment allows you to take part in once you are done with your workday.

- **Are you prevention-focused or promotion-focused?** Motivation is a powerful thing, and research has shown that most people belong to one of two very different motivational types: they either play to win or play not to lose. There isn't one type that is better than the other; both are necessary for an innovative yet consistent work environment. However, the two different types react very differently in the workplace.

  The promotion-focused person is the type who is inspired by the goal of making new gains. They play to win and are driven by optimism and praise. They are more creative, innovative and more willing to take risks in order to make those gains. They are also more likely to make mistakes and not think things completely through.

  The prevention-focused person is the type who is more inspired by the goals of playing it safe and maintaining consistency. They play not to lose and are driven by criticism and the looming threat of failure. They are more careful and accurate in order to succeed in not losing ground. They are also more likely to be overly cautious and may risk becoming stuck in old ways while their field evolves around them.

  As you can imagine, if a manager and a subordinate or members of a team have different motivational types, there is a potential for a lot of miscommunication, frustration and misunderstanding. The book *Focus: Use Different Ways of Seeing the World for Success and Influence* by Heidi Grant Halvorson, PhD and E. Tory Higgins, PhD is a great reference which can help you learn more about these types and how to navigate the differences.

Other helpful self-knowledge resources include:
- Meyers Briggs Personality Type (http://www.myersbriggs.org)
- *The Highly Sensitive Person,* by Elaine N. Aron, PhD
- *StrengthsFinder 2.0,* by Tom Rath

Other Potential Causes of Stress

There are other aspects of life that may also be contributing a significant amount of stress to the contents of your "bucket." For example, poverty and bias are two potential sources of stress that can increase your chances of burnout. If you are experiencing financial insecurity or are someone who is subjected to social bias, you may need to balance out your burnout resiliency by building up your other areas.

How about the other stressful events you've experienced recently? Have you experienced a divorce, had a death in the family or gotten into an accident? In Chapter 5 you were asked to find your score on the Holmes and Rahe Life Stress Inventory. This stress scale has been shown repeatedly to predict one's risk for a "health breakdown" over the next two years. Thomas Holmes and Richard Rahe initially developed the inventory in 1967 by studying the medical records of over 5,000 medical patients.

Their key insights were that both positive and negative events add stress, and that the stress occurs both in adapting to the stressful event and then in regaining a new equilibrium. Depending on your own personal circumstances, you may well rate the relative stress levels of these life events somewhat differently (and of course not all stressful events are listed on the scale!) Nevertheless, the Holmes and Rahe Life Stress Inventory has been repeatedly tested over the years, and found to be useful in men, in women, and in children (though the relative ratings do change a little for kids). The Inventory has also been tested in a wide range of cultures and been translated into a wide variety of languages.

Addiction Hurts

If you or someone you love is suffering with an addiction, there is help available for you. It is widely recognized that stress is a significant risk factor in the development of addiction. Stress can also increase the rate of addiction relapse.

You may rationalize it as a few drinks to "wind down" after a stressful day, but is that all it is? Chronic stress can make you far more vulnerable to addictive behaviors. It can alter the structure of your brain, your desires and impulses, and affect the way you respond to distress.

Addiction comes in many shapes and sizes. Some people become addicted to shopping, drugs, sex, eating, or even video games. So if you've been in a stressful situation that has led you to burnout and has also led you to addiction, you aren't alone.

Addiction is a disease, a disease for which there is a cure. Don't do this alone — find help! If you work in a place with an Employee

Assistance Program (EAP), use this service to help you find the best services in your area. You can also ask your health care provider or search online for addiction help in your area. Here are common helpful resources to get you started:

- Alcoholics Anonymous: www.aa.org
- National Institutes on Drug Abuse: https://www.drugabuse.gov/publications/principles-drug-addiction-treatment-research-based-guide-third-edition/resources

Assess for Abuse

If you are in an abusive situation, there is no doubt that you are experiencing a great deal of stress because of it. Are you safe in your personal and work environment? Are you safe in your personal and work relationships? Unfortunately, abusive relationships are all too common. People who end up in abusive situations or relationships, whether personal or professional, often don't realize it. They are commonly people who do not think of themselves as victims. It just may be that, for one reason or another, they put up with inappropriate behavior for so long that they didn't notice when it crossed the line into abusive, or even illegal behavior. However, if you find yourself in an abusive situation, it is best to get out of it. The cost to your health and safety just aren't worth it.

There are many signs that you may be in an abusive situation: If you are feeling constantly belittled or controlled, if there's lots of yelling or constant criticism, if you are excluded from group activities, if you are the subject of lies or gossip, or even if you feel physically ill before entering into the situation, you may be in an abusive situation.

In the workplace, there are many common legal lines that people often don't recognize are being crossed. Several include abuse of wage and hour laws. For instance, hourly employees must be given breaks of specific length at specific intervals. Supervisors who force employees to perform work duties before or after they clock in are doing something called "wage theft." There should be a poster available at your workplace that reviews these laws. If not, they are easily found online if you search "your rights under wage and hour laws."

Bullying of employees may not necessarily be illegal, but harassment based on a protected characteristic, such as gender, race, age, sexual orientation, religion or national origin *is* illegal.

Also, "retaliation is the most frequently alleged basis of discrimination in the federal sector and the most common discrimination finding in federal sector cases." Employers and supervisors are not allowed to discriminate, harass, or otherwise punish an employee in retaliation to their action in an Equal Employment Opportunity (EEO) issues, such as being witness in an EEO lawsuit, communicating with a supervisor about discrimination, resisting sexual advances or intervening to protect others, requesting accommodation of a disability or for religious practice or asking about salary information to uncover potentially discriminatory wages.

Resources for Help

The good news is that there are resources to help. If you have any doubts at all, please seek advice from someone who can help you sort through these issues. Your company's HR professional should have resources to help you, but if you aren't satisfied with the answers you receive there, please continue to seek help.

For personal relationships, the National Domestic Violence Hotline is 1-800-799-7233, 1-800-787-3224 (TTY), or www.thehotline.org.

To find out more about workplace safety issues, the Occupational Safety and Health Administration number is 1-800-321-6742, www.osha.gov. For wage and hour issues, contact the United States Department of Labor Wage and Hour Division at 1-866-487-9243 or www.dol.gov/whd/contact_us.htm.

If you feel you've been discriminated against, you can contact the US Equal Employment Opportunity Commission at 1-800-669-4000 or www.eeoc.gov. There may also be specific laws in your state that protect you, so please contact your state's department of labor for that information.

Chapter Nine

Community: Reconnect, Ask for Help, Get Perspective

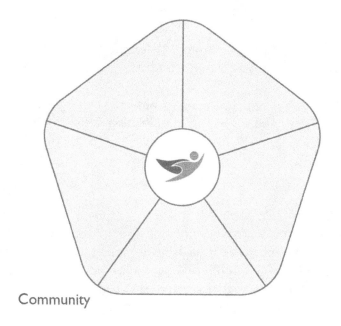

Community

"Call it a clan, call it a network, call it a tribe, call it a family. Whatever you call it, whoever you are, you need one."
—*Jane Howard*

Quick check in:
**Do you feel connected with a community of people who care about
you and share your values? Do you interact enough with them?**

Elements of Community

The following list includes elements of your sense of community. When you have a strong sense of community, including positive communication, humor, shared values and a sense of teamwork, it can help mitigate the stress of your work and other responsibilities. In addition, members of your community can help you by lending a hand or an outside perspective when you need it the most. Burnout can be incredibly isolating, but a strong connection with the members of your community can help protect you from that isolation.

Connection to community	Personal relationship	Ability to ask for help	Outside perspective
Sense of teamwork	Caring for/from	Delegating to others	Positivity ratio
Relationship with boss	Communication skills	Conflict resolution skills	Coworkers who vent
Respect			

Overall Community Goal

Identify the members of your community who provide you with the greatest sense of camaraderie, friendship or support. If connections like these are missing from your life, seek out connections with like-minded people through professional or social organizations. Interactions with your community are crucial for protecting you against burnout.

Where to Start

1. **Review** the Community elements listed above. (It may be helpful to review your answers from the Community section of the Burnout Shield Assessment.)
2. Put a **check mark** by each element of Community that you are currently managing well.
3. **Underline** each element of Community that you'd like to improve.
4. Of those that you underlined, **circle** any that you are most motivated or feel most equipped to change right now. As you do this,

consider whether or not you have the required skills, necessary resources, or control over your schedule, etc.

5. **Rebuild with positive changes.** Fill in the **To Do List** below with your plan for positive changes. *Note: You may want to wait to fill this out until after you've read the rest of the chapter.*

   Start where you have indicated you are the most motivated. We recommend that you start with one small change that is easy to incorporate into your daily schedule. Once you've been successful with that positive change, acknowledge your accomplishment and then continue to add more positive changes to your daily routine.

6. **Expand your insight, knowledge and skill level:** As you read on, you'll learn more about the different areas of Community and how they impact your health and your ability to withstand burnout. We share some of our own stories and stories from the people that we've helped. You'll also find some additional resources and assessment tools that can help you become more familiar with aspects of Community.

   Considering how vast these topics are, this chapter is intended only as a guide to some elements of Community that are most directly related to your ability to withstand burnout. However, we encourage you to reach beyond this book. There are so many helpful Community resources out there, and they can be the doorway to a great deal of healing of strength.

Positive Changes

Here are some examples of positive changes you can make for the different elements of Community.

Connection to community
- Join your professional organization.
- Volunteer on a committee (as long as you have the energy and time to do this.)
- Join a community-based activity that also benefits one of your other Burnout Shield areas. For example, join a lunchtime walking group (Self-Care.)

Sense of teamwork; Relationship with boss; Respect
- Make a personal resolution to avoid office politics and gossip.

- Identify the preferred contact method and time of day for each member of your team.
- Acknowledge people when they are speaking to you.

Personal relationship; Caring for/from
- Actively work on your own happiness.
- Practice listening with the intent to understand, not fix.
- Learn to tell people how you are feeling and how they can help you in that moment.

Communication skills; Asking for help
- When communicating, LTPRV: Listen, Think, Pause, Respond and then Verify that you addressed the main issue.
- When asking for help, give specifics about what you need done, why it is needed and when you need it to be finished.
- Create a culture where help is freely requested and also given when needed.

Delegating to others
- Let go of the need to do everything yourself.
- Get to know the strengths and skills of others on your team so you can play to each person's.
- Thank people for accepting the responsibility for the tasks you delegate.

Conflict resolution skills; Outside perspective
- Encourage all parties involved to calm down before attempting resolution.
- Practice active listening by paying attention, asking questions and verifying that you understood what was said.
- Seek advice from someone you admire who has been through a similar situation in the past.

Positivity ratio; Coworkers who vent
- Say at least three positive comments for each negative one. Encourage others in your home and office to do this as well.
- Avoid venting or being exposed to the venting of others — this can be a very contagious way to spread burnout!

- If you must vent your frustrations, convert the process into the first step of a more healthy coping mechanism. You've identified the problem. Now what?

Community To-Do List

Positive Change I will try first:

_____

_____

_____

Positive Changes I am interested to try in the near future:

_____

_____

_____

Positive Changes I may incorporate someday, but will put aside until I've successfully incorporated the changes listed above:

_____

_____

_____

Community Results

Positive Changes that have made the greatest difference in my life:

_____

_____

_____

_____

Elements of Community that I tend to let slip when I am under stress:

_____

_____

_____

_____

Helpful Community reminder for myself the next time I'm under stress:

_____

_____

_____

_____

Community and Teamwork

It is common to feel isolated when you are burned out. It can be part of the cause that led you to burnout, or it could be the result of your burnout itself, specifically the second dimension of burnout: fatigue, **cynicism**, low self efficacy.

However, we urge you to fight this tendency! As you save yourself from burnout, reconnecting with groups of like-minded people will help you. It is good for your psyche to belong to a group, especially if you have shared goals and values. The more you can cultivate a sense of teamwork with the people around you, the more you will be able to share the burden of stress and collectively work together to achieve your goals.

If you are having trouble thinking of anyone you have anything in common with, we'll help you: for starters, you are one of millions who are feeling burned out! That's just a starting place.

Where can you find your "group," your "tribe?"

- Professional associations for almost every different profession
- Associations for groups within those groups, for example: women engineers or Jewish dentists
- Religious, ethnic or cultural heritage groups
- Physical activity groups, such as walking, bike riding, etc.
- Service organizations, which are voluntary, non-profit groups where members meet regularly to perform charitable work, such as Rotary, Kiwanis, Soroptimists and many, many others.
- If you are an entrepreneur or work in a field that depends on business networking, you could join your local Chamber of Commerce or one of the many excellent business networking groups.
- Groups for people who currently have, have recovered from, or are related to someone who has a specific illness.
- Groups for people who want to practice specific skills, such as nonviolent communication or mindfulness.
- Recreational groups for any type of recreation, including sports, game playing, sewing, scuba diving, you name it!
- Family groups, either within the members of your family or groups that connect your family to other families for social gatherings.

An internet search can help you locate resources and contact information for these groups. Meetup.com is an excellent resource for finding like-minded groups of people. Also, look to your local Parks and Recreation office for resources.

If you live in a small town and the groups you'd most like to belong to do not exist there, you may still be able to find a sense of camaraderie by connecting in other ways with these non-local groups. Membership, correspondence, newsletters and even virtual social events may help you reconnect with people in a meaningful way.

Maintain Participation in Social Events

As we've said before in this book, committed, dedicated, passionate go-getters often defer or omit many of their personal priorities, in order to devote their time and energy to their primary purpose. They often do this in the name of "efficiency," or "time management." In the short run, personal sacrifices are often necessary to achieve success. In the long run, or if done in too extreme a way, personal sacrifices can be devastating because they can lead straight into burnout.

One of the sacrifices we may routinely make is that of our social life. With the pressures of career, family and perhaps volunteer commitments, many of us let go get-togethers such as a night out with friends, poker night, or the Saturday neighborhood soccer game because we've classified them as "frivolous" or "unproductive."

While it is true that a night out with friends might not directly help you with your professional or personal goals, it may still have a valuable role to play in helping to prevent your burnout. One way to decide if a social event needs to stay in your life is to assess it with your Burnout Shield. For example: Dr. Marnie Loomis likes to tell the story of her Trivia Night decision.

Marnie: Trivia Night and the Burnout Shield

For years, I'd been meeting a group of good friends most Wednesday nights at a pub for Trivia Night. We'd drink beer, laugh hard, and participate in team trivia contests. We all had our areas of strength; for instance, I am good at news-related trivia. We sometimes won, which was fun. But what was really fun was hanging out and laughing with these friends.

As my life got busier, I had more and more deadlines to meet and late nights at work. One particular night, I seriously considered not only skipping Trivia Night that evening, but also possibly stopping my participation altogether. But that didn't feel quite right. That's when I realized that I could assess my Trivia Night decision with the Burnout Shield. Here's what I came up with:

- **Self-Care.** The late night and the beer in the middle of the work week were not so great for my Self-Care, I had to admit. Count that as a negative.
- **Reflection & Recognition.** Well, I couldn't say that my core values were much affected by winning trivia contests. But the recognition and appreciation I got from my friends for helping the team, and the support I felt for the rest of our team both felt really good. Plus, we often caught up on each other's news before the game

started, and congratulated each other on any accomplishments of the week. Call this one a positive.

- **Capacity.** In the short run, yes, I'd free up some time and energy if I stopped going to Trivia Night. But I was pretty sure I'd miss the sense of camaraderie and the fun I had even more. I'm an extrovert, and I get sad and lonely if I don't often spend time with others. And sad and lonely is definitely not a productive state of mind for me. So, surprising myself, I had to put Capacity on the "mostly positive" side of the ledger.
- **Community.** Definitely positive, no question.
- **Coping Skills.** I enjoy Trivia Night, and I love my friends. That's all emotion-focused coping, which is appropriate to the situation. And I'm working out my decision about continuing with it by using the Burnout Shield to analyze it — that's problem-focused coping. So I've brought two major coping styles into play. Finally, I realized that I find myself in a good mood the day or two following every Trivia Night, which helps me cope with the stress at work. In terms of Coping Skills, definitely a positive!

A negative for Self Care, positive for Recognition, plus-minus for Capacity, and positives for Community and Coping Skills. Trivia Night wins, 3.5 out of 5!

I continue to keep my commitment to participate in weekly Trivia Nights whenever possible, because I'm secure in the knowledge that for me, it's a key to keeping burnout out of my life.

Communication and Motivational Style

Help your coworkers and your supervisor understand you better by letting them know your primary motivational focus. Are you promotion-focused or prevention-focused? Your primary motivational focus influences the way you act, what you value and how you act when you succeed or fail.

People with each type of focus are valuable. Successful teams are the ones that learn how to communicate effectively with each other. They learn to appreciate the abilities that both types have to offer.

You probably have both types of focus from time to time, but which is your main focus? Use the table below to find out.

Promotion-Focused Person		Prevention-Focused Person
Eager and willing to take chances	*or*	Vigilant and aim to avoid mistakes
Goals often centered on receiving recognition or some sort of reward	*or*	Goals often centered on responsibility and a successful prevention of loss
Concentrate on potential achievements, regret lost opportunities	*or*	Concentrate on staying safe and worry about what might go wrong
Play to win	*or*	Play not to lose
Work quickly	*or*	Work slowly and meticulously
Creative	*or*	Analytical
May seem optimistic, plan for the best-case scenario	*or*	May seem pessimistic, prepare for the worst-case scenarios
Comfortable trying new methods	*or*	Prefers tried and true methods
Will work harder when assured I am on target to reach a goal	*or*	Will work harder when I am told that they are below target but can catch up
Finished work is more prone to errors, less likely to have all details worked out	*or*	Finished work is thorough, accurate, carefully considered
Seek positive feedback and confirmation that I am trusted; loses steam without it	*or*	Uncomfortable with overly-cheerful praise, motivated by constructive criticism
Feel dejected or depressed when things go wrong	*or*	Feel worried or anxious when things go wrong

Table 9.1 Are you primarily promotion-focused or prevention-focused?

Communicating with the Team: What Motivates You? What Motivates Them?

Have you ever felt that the instructions and feedback you receive actually leave you feeling less motivated overall? Even when, objectively, your manager or colleague has said nothing wrong or objectionable? In our experience, this communication problem may revolve around mismatches in motivational style.

For example, the two of us usually find that our ideas are often synergistic and our tandem working sessions extremely productive. We both love science and research. We're both meticulous, cautious, and detail-oriented. We both get excited and energized by new ideas and grand concepts.

Yet, sometimes we'd come out of a session of working together with one or both of us feeling deflated, frustrated and even angry. When we learned about the book by Heidi Grant Halvorson and Tory Higgins, *Focus: Use Different Ways of Seeing the World for Success and Influence* (on whose work the quiz above is based) the two of us experienced an Ah-Ha moment.

We realized quickly that Dr. Marnie is usually promotion-focused. She's a visual and visionary thinker, highly creative, and finds herself energized by praise and goals that are phrased in aspirational language. She works well when deadlines are close and the pressure is on.

By contrast, Beth is usually prevention-focused. She thinks in words and concepts, rarely pictures. She's most motivated by constructive criticism, and is generally unmoved by lofty goals unless they are supported by closely-reasoned analysis. She usually prepares in advance, and dislikes the pressure of last-minute prep.

When we thought about our working meetings that did not go well, we realized that the problems nearly always stemmed from these previously unconscious differences in motivational style. Dr. Loomis would present her ideas with big flourish and excitement. Beth Genly would carefully poke holes in the ideas, probing for all the ways she felt they needed to be more airtight and structured. Dr. Loomis would lose energy for the ideas and feel sad or anxious or mad. Or, Beth would present a carefully detailed list of goals and sub-goals. Dr. Loomis would say, "Let's not worry about the details just yet, let's just go for it!" In response, Beth would feel deflated and unmotivated.

Now, when we hit one of these impasses, one of us will say, "Oh, Promotion!" or, "Ah-hah, Prevention!" Then we laugh and rephrase. Now that we are aware *why* we each feel differently in these situations, the mismatch in our styles doesn't derail us any more. In fact, we use this knowledge to delegate tasks to each other that we know would be much more fun for the other to do.

We run a motivational style exercise in live workshops where, instead of checking boxes on a list, we mark one side of the room blue (promotion-focused) and one side red (prevention-focused). We read each set of statements from the table aloud, and say, "If you identify with this one, stand on the blue side. If you identify with this next one, stand on the red side."

The results are often very interesting. This exercise allows each member of the team to see with whom they share a motivational style and with whom they do not. As we explain more about motivational styles and the frustrations or miscomprehensions that may arise out of team members not understanding their differences, we often see shared glances and nods of recognition. This is a fun exercise because it tends to reveal the hidden "code" behind a lot of workplace frustration.

For example, in one group of about 20 employees, about 12 people sorted themselves to the blue "promotion" side, while 8 of them went to the red "prevention" side. Even more interesting, people rarely switched sides as we read each new statement. After asking about their role in the company, we found that most of the top managers chose the blue side of the room and most of the people in jobs that involved quality control, accounting, and regulation-compliance chose the red side.

We then tried out different targeted motivational language on the two color groups. After reading each aloud, we asked each group how the statement made them feel.

Try it yourself. Imagine how you would feel if your boss or a colleague assigned you a task using one of the following statements:

"We've got an incredible team working on some exciting new ideas. This time, we are going to blow away last quarter's top numbers. The productivity record will be ours for sure!"

Or

"Last quarter, we didn't make the numbers we hoped for, so let's figure out what stood in our way and make sure none of those roadblocks are in our way this time!"

It is likely that one of these statements may strike you as inspiring and the other is just as likely to leave you feeling deflated and perhaps even irritated, sad or angry. Studies have found that motivational style matters when it comes to productivity and outcomes. The motivational statement needs to match the style of the recipient in order to be effective. Studies involving students who are asked to complete complicated tasks, and athletes encouraged to do their best in a game, show that outcomes will improve when the motivational statement matches the recipient and will either have no effect or an actual negative effect if a mismatched motivational statement is used.

Would a brief discussion of motivational style with others on your team help smooth these unintentional miscues and improve communication?

Communication, Delegation and Conflict Resolution Skills

There are many books written about each of these topics. The bottom line is that these all are made up of learned skills. You don't have to be a natural in order to be effective. You can work at it!

Resources for Conflict Resolution

In order from most tactical to most strategic, Thomas Cox, director of Becoming a Best Boss Training & Coaching, recommends these books (each with its own key lesson):

- Runde, Craig E., and Tim A. Flanagan. *Developing Your Conflict Competence: A Hands-on Guide for Leaders, Managers, Facilitators, and Teams.* Vol. 152. John Wiley & Sons, 2010. (Provides a model of destructive vs constructive conflict, and a vital shared language for discussing conflicts.)
- Patterson, Kerry. *Crucial conversations: Tools for talking when stakes are high.* Tata McGraw-Hill Education, 2002. (Provides step-by-step guidance for how to face and have tough conversations while maintaining relationships.)
- Friedes, Peter E. *The 2R Manager: When to Relate, When to Require, and How to Do Both Effectively.* Jossey-Bass, 2002. (Coaching on the mindset needed to both maintain relationships while still requiring excellence from subordinates.)
- McLaren, Karla. *The language of emotions: what your feelings are*

trying to tell you. Boulder, CO: Sounds True, 2010. (Helps you understand all your emotions and gives you tools to manage them well and effectively.)

- Schnarch, David. *Intimacy and desire: Awaken the passion in your relationship.* Scribe Publications, 2010. (Gives you tools and a framework for managing conflict in a peer or intimate relationship; much of this generalizes to work.)
- Peck, Morgan Scott. *The road less travelled.* Random House, 2012. (Gives both a model and a rationale for how to find the internal strength to face conflict well, with a spirit of love of self and others.)

Ask for Help: The Mindset Shift

Many of us are more than happy to *give* help. But…ask for help? This may be the toughest challenge this book will pose for you.

Asking for help sometimes means:

- Admitting that you don't know something you feel you are supposed to know.
- Sharing that you are stuck or upset. At that moment you might even look like you are not 100% in control.
- Confessing that you need support.
- Facing the possibility that you may not get help, or it may not come in a form you want.

Last year, Beth had a day in which, she says, "I had my nose rubbed (gently) in all of the above realizations, and it brought me to a major mindset shift about asking for help."

See if any parts of Beth's Mindset Shift story resonate for you.

Beth: Mindset Shift Story

I was with my business mastermind group, made up of six entrepreneurial friends who gathered once a month to share ideas and brainstorm as we grew our businesses.

It was not my finest moment. Actually, I was just about in tears. I was feeling stuck and frustrated and even a bit hopeless. My friends were not responding to my upset with the loving warmth and support I had wanted and expected. In fact, they were annoyed.

I finally confronted them. (I'm still proud of myself for that.) I said,

"Why are you angry with me? Are you aware of how you're treating me?"

There was a short silence. I could see each of my friends taking a quick look inside their own heads and hearts. After a few minutes of calmer conversation, Tom was finally able to articulate the source of their annoyance.

"You won't listen," he said. "You sound like you don't want help, even as you're asking for it." They all nodded. Another brief silence.

"You deserve all the help you need," Tess said. Somehow, that message finally went in. I got it.

You deserve all the help you need.

At first, I didn't even realize that I got it. Right then, frankly, I was still feeling put upon and frustrated and annoyed right back at them. (Like I said, not my finest moment.)

But afterward, that statement rang like a bell through my days: I deserve all the help I need.

I enrolled in a speaker's marketing class. My sections of this book started pouring out of me. I enrolled in a book marketing class. I let Marnie know that certain sections of the book felt overwhelming to me—and they turned out to be topics she was pleased to write about. What a relief. Teamwork!

With all this support, my task-oriented soul could relax. Simply hanging out with my family and friends—an activity that has always made me a bit antsy—became a lot more fun for me. I could stop pushing quite so hard, because *I deserve all the help I need.*

In case this makes you think my life is now entirely drenched in rainbows and surrounded by dancing unicorns: Not so much. Asking for help is still hard for me. After a few weeks (weeks! Lucky me!) of basking in "I can ask for anything," I once again caught myself worrying that I was really supposed to be solving everything, all the time, on my own. But I *did* catch myself. So, after a little struggle, I was able let it in once again: *I deserve all the help I need.* It gets easier, the more I let myself repeat it.

Once again I caught myself feeling I was really supposed to be solving everything, all the time, on my own.

And so, in the best tradition of paying it forward, I offer this thought to you.

Can you let it in?

You deserve all the help you need.

Confronting Stigma and Getting Help

At that same teachers' conference we mentioned in Chapter 1, the conference where we asked attendees about burnout at work, another conversation came up frequently.

"Well, do you talk about burnout, share tips and strategies?"

"Oh no, never."

"Why do you think that is?"

"Well…I guess we're a little afraid that the person with burnout might be so miserable that they'd just explode and splatter it all over the rest of us."

As we said in Chapter 1, we've found this is a very common fear. We decided to ask for help from an expert, someone who deals with far more intense stigma than that attached to burnout.

Tara Rolstad runs a non-profit called Shattering Stigma, where she deals with the shame associated with mental illness. Tara speaks to many groups about opening dialogues and creating safe spaces for conversations around mental illness. We figured if anyone would know how to deal with feeling stymied by stigma, she would. She did not let us down.

Tara said, "First, it's important to name it for what it is. When you're facing a situation you may have previously had a lot of thoughts about, along the lines of "If that ever happened to me, I would…" having those potentially misinformed preconceptions doesn't change when you DO find yourself in that situation. If you always judged people harshly who found themselves overweight and out of shape, then those judgments are still harsh, initially, when you find yourself overweight and out of shape. If you or a loved one is facing a mental illness, you still have to work through your own assumptions about why it happened and what it means.

"So take the time to name it. Name the stigma or the shame you're feeling, because those feelings don't change when it's your own experience, until you examine it, own it, and get better information.

"Next, imagine yourself out of the situation. Imagine that it's happened instead to your best friend, or a loved one. What advice would you give them? Probably, you'd be compassionate and supportive to them, right? Be willing to give yourself the grace you would give to someone you care about who found themselves in this situation."

Beth replied, "That's great, Tara, but what do you do if you've dealt with your own stigma, but you're still afraid you're going to meet some negative judgments from the people around you?"

"Assume the worst," Tara said.

"Really?"

"Yes. Assume that they do have those judgments and preconceptions, and make plans for how you're going to deal with it. Practice what you'll say, calmly and firmly, if you happen to need to. And know that, by staying silent, you would be hurting not just yourself but other people. You may even be putting other people at risk. Just decide: If I get judged for this at work, or wherever, then I've told myself I deserve this, I'm worth this.

"Sometimes, if you're buried under that feeling of 'I can't ask for help' — break it down into really small baby steps, and start with the first one, even if you don't feel like it. There is a freedom to realizing that even if I don't feel like it, I can still do it anyway."

Tara went on, "When my three young nieces all came to live with me, and all three turned out to have PTSD and mental illness, that situation forced me into a deep understanding of my own inadequacy. That was a complicated, emotional situation, and my 'good mom' skills were not nearly enough to deal with it. I just *could not* handle that situation alone. I *had* to ask for help, or sink.

"That learning has stayed with me. Now that my mom's aging, in failing health, and losing her independence, I very quickly realized I couldn't handle that situation by myself either. Much more quickly than I might have in the past, I turned to 'OK, who can help me?'

"Also, I know that this is not wasted pain. The grief I am feeling now as I help my mom will make me able to help someone else down the road who is going through the same thing.

"I have learned that the quicker I ask for help, the easier and less painful it is to ask. And, finally, asking for help is a great role model. It makes it easier for the people watching you to give themselves permission to ask for help."

If you'd like to know more about Tara Rolstad's deeply moving story about foster-parenting her three nieces, and the unusual but powerful solution she found for her own stress, read the book she co-authored with Dave Mowry: *No, Really, We Want You to Laugh: Mental Illness and Stand Up Comedy: Transforming Lives.*

In a Nutshell: Asking for Help

Here's Tara Rolstad's steps to take if you're having trouble asking for the help you need, because of embarrassment or shame.

- Name it for what it is, a condition you might have harshly judged in the past, when you saw it in other people. Note if there is shame attached to this condition, for you. Feelings can change when they are faced and named.
- Next, imagine yourself out of the situation. Imagine that it's happened instead to your best friend, or a loved one. What advice would you give them?
- Assume some people may well make harsh judgments and negative comments. Practice what you will say, calmly and firmly.
- If the problem is overwhelming, break it down into baby steps, and start with the first one. Even if you don't feel like it, there's a freedom in doing it anyway.
- The quicker you ask for help, the easier and less painful it is to ask.
- Know that you are a role model. When you ask for help, it may make it easier for others to ask for the help they need.

Interactive: Ask for Help Worksheet

1. Name a problem, task or responsibility where you feel overwhelmed. An area in which you've been toughing it out on your own.

_____

_____

_____

2. If you expect negative comments on your need for help, what will you say, firmly and calmly?

_____

_____

_____

3. Does the problem need to be broken down into baby steps? Write them here:

_____

_____

_____

4. Who knows how to address part of this problem, and how will you ask for their assistance?

_____

_____

_____

The Secret to Finding a Mentor

Mentors offer perspective, knowledge and personal connections and introductions. There's an open secret about how to find a mentor: there's an art to asking someone to be your mentor. Without knowing this art, the interaction might not go well for you.

Jen Dziura of GetBullish says, (we know because she displayed exactly these words on a PowerPoint slide) "No one wants to be *asked* to be your goddamn mentor. It's creepy."

So we asked Susan Bender Phelps, principal of Odyssey Mentoring and author of the wonderful little book *Aspire Higher* how to ask for help from a prospective mentor. We started by quoting that Dziura comment to her.

Bender Phelps nodded. "You just don't walk up to a stranger and say, 'Will you be my mentor?' That *is* creepy," she said. "Instead, you approach someone you know and admire, with a request that sounds something like this." "You know, Jesse, you used to work as a nurse-midwife, and I'm just starting my first year in midwifery practice — I just got notified I passed my Boards! Would you mind having coffee with me, and talking about what your first year was like for you?"

"It's likely," Bender Phelps said, "Jesse would be flattered and pleased to chat. At the end of your coffee date, then you say, 'This has been lovely, and very useful. Would you mind if I called you in six months and let you know how it's going for me?' Jesse would likely say yes."

"Then what you do, " Bender Phelps continued, "is you call Jesse back in *three* months and say, 'I just had to call and let you know, I followed your advice on X and Y to the letter, and it has made a huge difference to me in this specific way,' and you explain the positive difference that following her advice made for you. Then you hang up. What you're doing, there, is you're wooing this person. And then, of course, you do call back at the six month mark as well.

"In the olden days, an older man would spot a young man in the company, and say to himself, 'that guy reminds me of my younger self,' and he would take the younger man under his wing. He'd introduce him to important people, make sure he got on certain committees or projects, and encourage him to join key organizations. The word 'mentor' was never spoken. That was just how the old boy network worked. Women [and, we would add, people of color] don't have that. In this day and age, we still don't have that. So we need to build it.

"And often we may choose to have more than one mentor. For instance, we might call one person when we need business advice, and another when we need an upgrade on our technical skills.

"And while I strongly believe that mentorships are, and ought to be, volunteer relationships, it is also true that both parties get a lot of benefit. I like to quote the Catalyst study that showed that people who mentor rise higher and earn more than their colleagues who don't. Up to $25,000 a year more!"

So there you have it, from a mentorship expert. Build your mentorship relationship, one step at a time.

Ask For Help

Whether your burnout is mild or severe, you *can* feel better. We want you to feel better, and so do your colleagues and your family. Let it in: *You deserve all the help you need.*

Increase Positivity and Collegiality

Negative statements, especially when they are accurate descriptions of painful or adverse circumstances, are, of course, very important to effective human function. Without being able to acknowledge and clearly assess difficulties, our growth and progress would be impossible. In addition, our brains are more attuned to threats than pleasant events; we get more emotional "charge" out of a negative event than a similar positive one (for example, studies comparing the gain or loss of $20 showed the loss to be a more intense emotional experience for almost everyone.)

Being positive, while generally less intense, turns out to be critical for healthy functioning as well. Luckily, positivity is a learnable skill.

For a while, researchers were excited to think they could identify what the exact ratio of positive comments ought to be for healthy, productive communities. It was thought that we should aim for no less than 3 positive comments to every negative one. Later, an upper limit was also proposed: a ratio of more than 7 (or perhaps 11) positive comments to every negative one was felt to be the Pollyanna limit. (Pollyanna was the central character of a children's book published in 1913 as well as a 1960 Disney movie based on the book; the name has come to mean "an excessively cheerful or optimistic person.")

Lately, these positivity ratios have come into question — perhaps it was just too much to hope that we could have a hard and fast rule that would apply in all situations. The science behind the underlying principle is robust, however. A pioneering researcher in positive psychology, Barbara Frederickson, PhD, stated in a recent article on this subject, "Little by little, micro-moments of positive emotional experience, although fleeting, reshape who people are by setting them on trajectories of growth and building their enduring resources for survival." In other words, Dr. Frederickson was saying that just about every little bit of positivity helps us grow into stronger, kinder, more resilient human beings.

Frederickson concluded, "The data say that when considering positive emotions, more is better, up to a point, although this latter caution may be limited to self-focused positive emotions. The data also say that when considering negative emotions, less is better, down to a point. Negativity can either promote healthy functioning or kill it, depending on its contextual appropriateness and dosage relative to positive emotions."

Some interesting burnout research translated this concept of positive speech into "expressions of civility and respect" and took it into many

Veteran's Administration facilities. Dr. Michael Leiter developed a team who published a series of impressive studies on the CREW process: Civility, Respect and Engagement at Work. When VA departments (including managers) voluntarily decide to engage with defining civility and respect for their region and their institution, and then implement the concepts their way, they have "...shown significant improvements to recruitment, retention, attendance, wellbeing and customer service. Not to mention the time and aggravation saved for managers and employees caught up in negative work situations."

In describing CREW initiatives, Dr. Leiter and his team said, "There are good reasons to improve collegiality.

"An environment of civility and respect is a thing of value in itself. It also provides a vital resource for workplace health and productivity. When present, it brings happiness and fulfillment. Its absence drives people away. For businesses that depend upon attracting and inspiring high quality personnel, a civil, respectful work culture provides an essential infrastructure.

"Although strict, zero-tolerance policies are understandable and perhaps effective to combat abusive or violent behavior at work, these policies in themselves are not sufficient to inspire collegiality. Instead, positive expressions of camaraderie and respect come from the heart. A genuine and convincing expression of respect arises from within an appreciation of the quality and potential of another person."

Interactive: The Positivity Ratio

Research has found that the ratio of positive to negative comments in a work or home environment has a tremendous impact on the level of productivity.

What do you believe is the current ratio of positive to negative comments in your environments?

_____

_____

_____

How can you work to maintain a ratio of roughly 3:1–7:1 of positive comments to negative comments in your interactions?

_____

_____

_____

Avoid People Who Are Venting

You've spent most of this chapter reading about ways you can connect with other people. One important thing to avoid is too much exposure to people who deal with their frustrations by simply venting them. As we've said before, venting quickly spreads burnout from person to person. Yes, expressing frustrations may be necessary, but it can add to your stress if it goes on without any sort of next step to do something about the frustration or the source of it.

Choose to spend your time among people whom you admire for their ability to deal with stress. Those skills can be contagious, too!

Chapter TEN

Coping Skills: Rethink Your Reactions

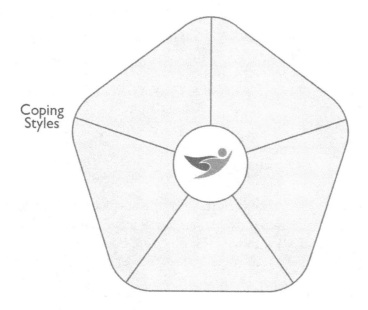

Coping
Styles

"The green reed which bends in the wind is stronger than the
mighty oak which breaks in a storm."
—*Confucius*

Quick check in:
Are your coping strategies helping you?
Or are they adding to the overall problem?

Elements of Coping Skills

The following list includes elements of Coping Skills. How do you respond to stress? While this part of yourself may run on autopilot, you have a lot to gain by making a conscious effort here. For most of us, coping is a learned skill, although part of it depends on your genetics and innate personality traits. This explains why some people are naturally able to handle whatever life throws at them.

Pause before react	Processing negative emotions	Use of humor	Hobby as response to stress
Brief Breaks	Seek advice of others	The Bright Side	Alcohol, drugs, smoking
Multitasking	Allow others to help	Exercise to manage stress	Limit venting
Perception of control	Personal Practices		

But you don't have to be *born* resilient to actually *be* resilient. Just like cooking, judo or riding a bike, you can practice and learn! There are many ways to develop these skills, which are imperative for saving yourself from burnout. Your response to stress determines how stress will affect you.

Overall Coping Skills Goal

You can change the way you respond to stress and learn to minimize the damage by coping effectively.

Where to Start

1. **Review** the Coping Skills elements listed above. (It may be helpful to review your answers from the Coping Skills section of the Burnout Shield Assessment.)
2. Put a **check mark** by each element of Coping Skills that you are currently managing well.

3. **Underline** each element of Coping Skills that you'd like to improve.

4. Of those that you underlined, **circle** any that you are most motivated or feel most equipped to change right now. As you do this, consider whether or not you have the required skills, necessary resources, or control over your schedule, etc.

5. **Rebuild with positive changes.** Fill in the **To Do List** below with your plan for positive changes. *Note: You may want to wait to fill this out until after you've read the rest of the chapter.*

   Start where you have indicated you are the most motivated. We recommend that you start with one small change that is easy to incorporate into your daily schedule. Once you've been successful with that positive change, acknowledge your accomplishment and then continue to add more positive changes to your daily routine.

6. **Expand your insight, knowledge and skill level:** As you read on, you'll learn more about the different areas of Coping Skills and how they impact your health and your ability to withstand burnout. We share some of our own stories and stories from the people that we've helped. You'll also find some additional resources and assessment tools that can help you become more familiar with aspects of Coping Skills.

   Considering how vast these topics are, this chapter is intended only as a guide to some elements of Coping Skills that are most directly related to your ability to withstand burnout. However, we encourage you to reach beyond this book. There are so many helpful Coping Skills resources out there, and they can be the doorway to a great deal of healing of strength.

Positive Changes

Here are some examples of positive changes you can make for the different elements of Coping Skills:

Pause before reacting; Brief breaks; Multitasking

- Before reacting to something stressful, pause and take a deep breath.
- Take brief diversion breaks to help to improve your long-term focus and productivity.

- Take the multitasking self-test to see if you are one of the rare 2% who is able to multitask efficiently.

Perception of control; Flexible thinking
- Exercise control in the areas where you do have it, even the small areas.
- Notice your language and self-talk patterns. Are you giving away your power? For example, saying "I can't," when you mean "I don't want to" or "This isn't my highest priority."
- Ask others, *"Why* do you think that?" rather than, "Why do you think *that?"*

Seek advice from others; Allow others to help; Personal practices
- Create a relationship with a person or group of people who have experienced a similar experience or who share your personal values (mentor, support group, professional network, religious or spiritual group.)
- Recognize that accepting help from others is a smart use of available resources, not a weakness.
- Ask those around you *how,* not *if,* they can help you.

Humor; Looking at the bright side
- Discover the type of humor you enjoy and immerse yourself in it
- Allow yourself to smile or laugh at jokes told by others.
- There is almost always a bright side, even if it is just the chance to learn from a mistake.

Hobby as a response to stress; Exercise to manage stress
- Choose a stress-relieving hobby that simultaneously benefits another area of your Burnout Shield.
- Recognize that participation in hobbies can be a mechanism of self-soothing. Is this how you are using yours, or have they become a new, additional sources of stress?
- Find enjoyable ways to incorporate movement into your daily schedule.

Limiting venting; Avoiding alcohol, smoking, drugs

- If you must vent, make it productive. Think of solutions or consider keeping a stress diary, which can help you track stress patterns.
- Avoid those who regularly vent their frustrations. Researchers have called venting a burnout "contagion," in other words, a way for burnout to spread from person to person.
- When you are under stress, limit or eliminate your use of alcohol, smoking or recreational drugs. Get help if necessary.

Coping Styles To-Do List

Positive change I will try first:

_____

_____

_____

Positive changes I am interested to try in the near future:

_____

_____

_____

Positive changes I may incorporate someday, but will put aside until I've successfully incorporated the changes listed above:

_____

_____

_____

Coping Styles Results

Positive changes that have made the greatest difference in my life:

_____

_____

_____

Elements of Coping Skills that I tend to let slip when I am under stress:

_____

_____

_____

Helpful Coping Skills reminder for myself the next time I'm under stress:

_____

_____

_____

Give Yourself a Fighting Chance

Here's the thing about coping: It is really easy to let yourself run on autopilot. In this chapter, we are going to ask you to pause and think about which coping mechanisms you are actively using. If you've gotten this far in life, you've likely developed a good collection of different coping techniques, but are you sure you are currently using the best technique for your given situation?

It's very easy to slip into a coping pattern that has worked for you in the past, but if you are dealing with burnout, it probably means you are in a high-stress environment filled with the type of stressful "mismatches" (see Chapter 2) that can drive you into burnout. In this chapter, we will review some of the basics about the different coping mechanisms so that you can carefully choose the most effective coping techniques for your specific situation and give yourself a fighting chance.

Your Personal Warning Signs in Action

In Chapter 3, we asked you to compile a list of your personal warning signs. This is where that list can come in handy. If you notice yourself doing any of the things on your list, stop and consider whether it is time to reevaluate your situation and find a better response.

Interactive: The Frog in the Pot

The old anachronistic metaphor about the "frog in the pot" speaks to this tendency we have, to be blind to change in our environment when it happens gradually. *If you put a frog into a hot pot, it will jump right out, but if you put a frog into a cold pot and then slowly heat it up, the frog will eventually let itself be heated to death.* Poor little frog.

Why doesn't the metaphorical frog save itself in both scenarios if it has the skills to do so? Because the frog, like most people, doesn't notice the gradual change. It continues to deal with the stress of the heat around it until it is overcome.

Have you remained in a situation that has become unbearable? Consider the following questions:

- Is your situation is the same as it was when you started, or has it gradually gotten worse?
- Was this initially supposed to be a temporarily stressful situation, but so far, hasn't relented?
- Is it reasonable to think that anyone would be able to handle the situation that you find yourself in now?

If you answered yes to any of these things, it may be time for a coping technique reevaluation.

An Overview of Coping Skills

Good vs. Bad

In general, one particular coping technique is not necessarily considered "bad" or "good." It depends on which technique is most appropriate for the situation. How do you know which is best? A big thing to consider is how much control you have over the cause of the stress. Another consideration is whether or not you currently have the resources to deal with the cause of the stress.

That being said, there are coping techniques that tend to cause more harm than good, such as turning to alcohol or drugs, denying, blaming others or emotionally disengaging from a situation. We strongly urge you to evaluate your coping responses and look for whether or not you are helping yourself or causing yourself more harm.

Problem-focused vs. Emotion-focused Coping Skills

Coping techniques can be split into two different major types, problem-focused and emotion-focused. Problem-focused coping aims to do something about the cause of the stress. Emotion-focused coping aims to bring you a sense of comfort when you are exposed to the stress.

The benefit of problem-focused coping is that you might actually resolve the cause of your stress and therefore eliminate it or at least change it in the long run. The downside is that it requires you to initially take on more work to do so. Another downside is that if you don't actually have control over the cause of the stress, or if you don't have all the resources (including time and energy), you might be fighting a battle that you have no chance to win.

The benefit of emotion-focused coping is that it lessens the negative impact of stress on your mind and body, which can help you to withstand the stress for longer periods of time. The downside is that it doesn't do anything about the cause of your stress, so you could potentially have to continue dealing with the stress indefinitely. If you are in a situation where you actually have control over the cause of your stress but you are only using emotion-focused coping, you may be exposing yourself to unnecessary long-term stress, which will decrease your ability to take on additional stress in the future.

For those of you who are visual learners, we created a flow chart that suggests how to choose between emotion-focused or problem-focused coping skills.

The Burnout Solutions Coping Methods Selection Tool

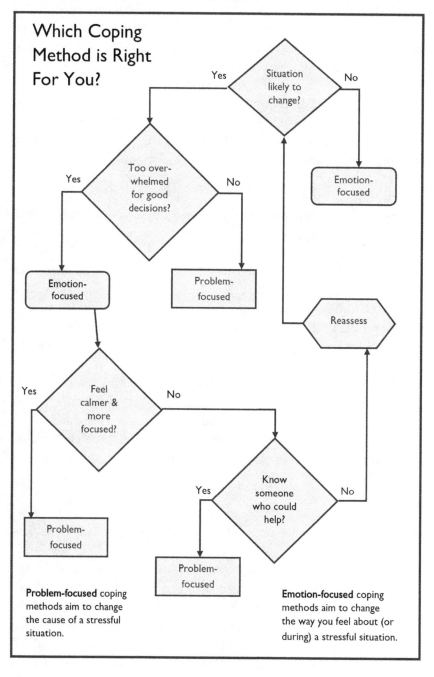

Which Coping Method is Right For You?

Situation likely to change?
Yes → Too over-whelmed for good decisions?
No → Emotion-focused

Too over-whelmed for good decisions?
Yes → Emotion-focused
No → Problem-focused

Emotion-focused → **Feel calmer & more focused?**
Yes → Problem-focused
No → Know someone who could help?

Know someone who could help?
Yes → Problem-focused
No → Reassess

Reassess

Problem-focused coping methods aim to change the cause of a stressful situation.

Emotion-focused coping methods aim to change the way you feel about (or during) a stressful situation.

Flexible Thinking

Flexible thinking is a benefit when it comes to coping with stress. If you see flexibility as weakness, consider which is stronger: the mighty oak that breaks in the storm or the reed that bends and survives. Flexible thinking can be represented by your ability to be flexible as you consider different types of solutions, unlearn the old way of doing things, understand the motivations of others, switch gears and think of a problem from a whole new perspective or even flexibility with what you consider to be a "win." Flexible thinking can give you a significant advantage when coping with stress.

Emotional Competence

When you are dealing with strong emotions, it can be difficult to steer yourself to the best possible coping technique for the situation. In order to train physicians to be able to manage the intense internal emotions, external situations and relationships involved in their everyday work lives, Loma K Flowers, MD, Clinical Professor of Psychiatry at the University of California San Francisco, developed a pragmatic training course for medical students that involved the following 10 Step feeling management protocol that combined "The Big Four": feelings, thinking, judgment and action (printed with permission).

I found this tool to be so helpful that I not only incorporated it into the classes I taught, but also kept copies of her article in my office to hand out to students, colleagues and alumni when they came to my office struggling with interpersonal conflict or making emotionally challenging decisions. I even brought a copy home for my children to use, and we put up on our fridge among the magnets, artwork, and other helpful resources.

A 10-step feeling management protocol: coordinating "The Big Four": feelings, thinking, judgment and action

1. Time out. When an event or situation occurs, pause while you complete steps 2–5. (An "event" can be examination anxiety, alcohol/drug abuse, family issue, academic challenge, safe sex concerns, need for an important decision, noticeable stress, etc.) This seems simple, but many problems derive from impulsive responses that preclude thinking or reflection about consequences.
2. Analyze what happened, i.e., examine the whole story, in chrono-

logical order, distinguish cause and effect, include feelings. Journaling helps here.

3. Name all your feelings as precisely as you can.

4. Sort your feelings into relevant, anachronistic and irrelevant, i.e. dragging in the kitchen sink.

5. Face all your feelings. Process them by exploring, examining and experiencing them without acting on them. This process can be facilitated by crying, journaling and talking to an appropriate person.

6. Choose the best result for now and later. Use good judgment and attend to relevant feelings.

7. Plan how to make that "best result" happen. Think carefully and be realistic. Set timelines. Enlist support from appropriate friends, colleagues, faculty, peers and professionals.

8. Follow your plan and nothing but your plan, but do follow your plan. Act.

9. Evaluate your results: examine feelings, what worked, what didn't and why.

10. Accept the results and move on. As needed, cycle back to Step 1, time out, with the modified or new situation.

Perception of Control and Learned Helplessness

The concept of locus of control addresses your assumptions about the responsibility for good and bad events that happen in your life. People's locus of control tends to be either predominantly internal (due to own actions, motivations, competencies) or external (due to luck, chance, others who are more powerful.)

Research has shown that people with an internal locus of control are more likely to perceive workplace demands as opportunities, not threats. They are more likely to choose problem-focused rather than emotion-focused coping techniques because they have more confidence that they can have a positive impact. In contrast, people with an external locus of control tend to become more stressed by workplace issues and report higher rates of immune system dysfunctions and related illnesses due to stress.

You can work to change your sense of locus of control. This is especially important in cases of learned helplessness. Learned helplessness can occur if you have been in a situation where you have suffered from uncontrollable bad events. If these events were severe enough or the experience was repeated often enough, you can develop a perceived lack of control, which can lead to a generalized behavior of lack of control.

The problem with learned helplessness is that people allow themselves to be hurt or stressed when they normally wouldn't allow this. They have been conditioned to forget that they actually have the power to protect themselves.

If you think you are stuck in a state of learned helplessness, exercises to increase your sense of control over anything in your environment can have positive impacts on your wellbeing. For an extreme example, patients who had been having difficulty dealing with the news that they had terminal conditions became more alert, more active, and happier when they were engaged in controlling aspects of their surroundings, such as the lights, music and menu choices.

How to Escape a Sense of Learned Helplessness
- Notice your language and self-talk.
- Phase out phrases like "I have no choice, I can't..." and replace with "I choose not to..." or "I don't like my choices, but I will..."
- Think of someone you admire. Consider what they might do if they were in your same situation.
- Review your options.
- Identify the areas in your situation where you do have control.
- Be aware that you have a choice.

It is also possible to have too much control. If you feel like you have too many choices, this can have its own negative impact. This is referred to as the tyranny of choice. In general, breaking options down into smaller groups, especially groups of three, can help to break up this sense of being overwhelmed.

Common Examples (Not All Good) of Coping Reactions
All of these things are examples of different coping reactions, but **not all of them are necessarily healthy or helpful.** You may have been doing some of these things but may not have recognized that they were a response to stress.

Active coping
- Take additional action to try to get rid of the problem.
- Do what has to be done, one step at a time.
- Drink caffeinated drinks or eat sugary snacks to give me the energy to continue working.

Planning
- Make a plan of action.
- Think about how you might best handle the problem.

Suppression of competing activities
- Focus on dealing with this problem, and if necessary let other things slide a little.
- Put aside other activities in order to concentrate on this.

Restraint coping
- Force yourself to wait for the right time to do something.
- Make sure not to make matters worse by acting too soon.

Seeking social support for instrumental reasons
- Ask people who have had similar experiences what they did.
- Talk to someone who could do something concrete about the problem.

Seeking social support for emotional reasons
- Talk to someone about how you feel.
- Try to get emotional support from friends or relatives.

Positive reinterpretation and growth
- Look for something good in what is happening.
- Learn something from the experience.
- Use humor.

Acceptance
- Be aware of what happens and can accept it without judgment.
- Learn to live with it.

Turning to religion
- Try to find comfort in your religion.
- Seek God's help.

Focus on and venting of emotions
- When you feel a lot of emotional distress and you find myself expressing those feelings a lot.
- Spend time in the company of others who focus on and vent their frustrated emotions.
- Have emotional outbursts toward others.

Denial
- Pretend that it hasn't really happened.
- Act as though it hasn't even happened.

Blaming others
- Be quick to show how others were to blame and it wasn't my fault.

Behavioral disengagement
- Just give up trying to reach your goal.
- Reduce the amount of effort you are putting into solving the problem.
- Try to avoid feeling negative emotions because they're overwhelming.

Mental disengagement
- Turn to work or other substitute activities to take your mind off things.
- Feel numb or try to avoid feeling your negative emotions because they're overwhelming.
- Fail to notice if I become injured or get sick.

Alcohol-drug disengagement
- Drink alcohol or take drugs, in order to think about it less.

Now that you've had the chance to identify some of your helpful and not-so-helpful coping reactions, take this opportunity to ask yourself:

Is this the best coping reaction for me at this time? It this causing more harm than good? Is it time to find a new way to cope?

Coping Skills Techniques in Action

Reframing, or "Seeing the Bright Side"
Human beings naturally interpret their experiences in the light of their own particular stories and beliefs. It happens in less than the blink of an eye, and we are often unaware that we have sent the "raw data" of our experiences through such a comprehensive filter.

A terrific low-effort way to reduce stress is to become aware that you use your own beliefs and stories to frame your understanding. Once you are aware of how you frame your "internal narrative," you are also able to modify the frame. Reframing in this way often soothes raw emotions and allows in new perspectives and solutions. It is most effective when you make not just a logical shift, but also an emotional one.

Often, talking it out without another person adds depth and power to this technique. Ask a trusted friend or mentor to help you play with your own internal script.

Flip the Script
Carter McNamara, a business consultant, lists a number of useful ways you can try shifting your perspective, including:
- **Shift from passive to active.** For example, if your statement is "I really doubt that I can do anything about this," you might reframe it as, "What is one small step that I might take?"
- **Shift from negative feeling to positive feeling.** For example, you might flip "I don't want to work on that now because it makes me feel angry," into, "What small part of that might I work on for now, that might even leave me feeling a bit calmer?"
- **Shift from past to future.** For example, if your thought is, "I've never been good at public speaking," you might respond, "If I imagined myself to be successful at public speaking, how would I be speaking that would be successful?" Another sometimes-useful version of this reframe is, "If I did know the answer to this, what would I know?" (Also, if you find yourself using the words "never" or "always" as you are framing a thought about your own or others' behavior, that thought is an excellent candidate for reframing.)

- **Shift from future to past.** For example, if your dilemma is, "I can't seem to get started on achieving this goal," you might respond, "Has there been a time in the past when I achieved a goal? What did I do back then to be successful? How might I use that approach now?"
- **Shift from a liability to an asset.** In other words, ask, "What's good about this?" For example, your response to "I'm such a perfectionist," might be "How might being a perfectionist help in me in my job and life, though?"
- **Shift from victimization to empowerment.** A classic example is the thought, "That always seems to happen to me." You might respond, "I wonder if I even do that to myself, somehow? If so, is there something about that I could change?"
- **Shift from "me" to "we."** Ask, how does this affect all of us rather than just me? For this shift, you might flip "That always seems to happen to me," into "That happens to a lot of us. Who in the group could I ask to address that issue with me?"

Here's an example of how these kind of reframing techniques can work. On New Year's Eve, one of our advisees shared her distress on Facebook this way:

Friend: *I feel bad and lonely because I'm barely talking to anyone. I'm barely talking to anyone because I only have the energy to really hold one conversation at a time (online). I don't have the energy because I spent over a weekend around too many people talking a lot. Oh, vicious cycle.*

We talked about the strategy of **reframing** to help her feel better and less stressed. In this case, spending 5 minutes **playing with the basic assumptions** expressed in our advisee's initial post allowed Beth to suggest half a dozen other ways to understand the same facts. Here is the rest of our Facebook conversation:

Beth Genly: *Re-frame?*

Friend: *Can you elaborate on this?*

Beth Genly: *Elaborate, sure. Your "vicious cycle" post is a clear and eloquent description of an introvert on overload. Wanting company, yet exhausted from too much company.*

A re-frame is a way to change your internal narrative or interpretation about a set of facts.

I can see several possibilities:

I learned something really important, and now I have a great story for teaching myself and others. Or,

I have many friends, I am so grateful, so today I can bask in glorious solitude. Or, moving out from the basics,

How can I create a delicious way to enjoy this day? Or, because sadness and loneliness is sometimes not so easily fought,

Now I am reminded of the obvious thing that these difficult emotions have to teach me: that I need connections, and I need to get them not all at once. What is a non-obvious further teaching that my reactions to my situation have to teach me? Or, [because many of her friends had already responded to her post with sympathetic and loving comments]

Look at how I used the energy of emotional exhaustion to reach out anyway on FB, and got LOVE back.

My point is, acknowledging and clearly naming how you feel right now allows you to honor your real feelings, and also to do some re-constructing of your story to try out some ways of finding hope and solace, too....That was pretty elaborate, yes?

Friend: *Have I told you recently that I love you? That was a fantastic elaboration, THANK YOU! I'm saving this to look at again when I need it in the future.<3*

Beth: *So glad I could help. You're welcome. Love you right back!*

Interactive: Practice Reframing

Can you think of still another way you could reframe our friend's distress? Write it here:

_____

_____

_____

To become familiar and comfortable with the various "flips," review your own reframing statement, as well as the ones from the New Year's scenario above. Which of the ways to "flip the script" might be in play for each of them? Choose from this list:

- **Shift from passive to active.**

- **Shift from past to future.**
- **Shift from future to past.**
- **Shift from a liability to an asset.**
- **Shift from victimization to empowerment.**
- **Shift from "me" to "we."**

Your reframed statement:

_____

The reframing strategy you used:

_____

I can see this situation as a teaching story.
    The reframing strategy used:

_____

I am grateful for my friends.
    The reframing strategy used:

_____

I will enjoy my glorious solitude today.
    The reframing strategy used:

_____

How can I enjoy the day as it is?
    The reframing strategy used:

_____

I am reminded that I need my friends.
    The reframing strategy used:

_____

I am reminded that I need to avoid overtaxing my introverted nature with too much socializing at once.

The reframing strategy used:

What else do my emotions have to teach me?

The reframing strategy used:

I am proud of reaching out on Facebook, even though I was tired.

The reframing strategy used:

Look at all these people who have expressed their love and care for me.

The reframing strategy used:

Another Reframing Strategy: The Work

Reframing is a powerful skill. Use it when you suspect that your internal narrative is keeping you stuck in difficult emotions, such as feeling hopeless, angry or sad.

Byron Katie developed another simple and powerful reframing system. She calls her system, simply, The Work. She's written several books about it, and has an extensive teaching website as well, called TheWork.com.

When reframing in this style, you start by writing down your distressing thought in the most emotional, blaming, nasty language you can drum up. Just in case you have any doubts about whether you're really supposed to express such unpleasantness to yourself, Katie calls her worksheet for this part the "Judge Your Neighbor" worksheet. Writing out your thoughts in this way allows you to surface your hidden suspicions and assumptions, which often unconsciously drive a lot of our distress. Once they are surfaced, you can examine them with clear eyes.

Next, in the Work, you ask these four questions about the Judge Your Neighbor statement you just wrote:

1. Is it true? (Yes or no. If no, move to 3.)
2. Can you absolutely know that it's true? (Yes or no.)
3. How do you react, what happens, when you believe that thought?
4. Who would you be without the thought?

Let's see how this works:

Let's say James is upset because a friend is not returning his phone calls. He is becoming fearful that the friendship is in jeopardy. Here's one way he might write out those fears in a negative, dramatic way, so he can do The Work:

"Janelle isn't calling me back because she's mad at me for something I said, and I'm not sure she likes me very much anyway."

Unpleasant thought! But James asks himself the first two questions. "Is it true? Can I absolutely know that it's true?"

He finds he really has no way to know the truth, since his whole thought involves a story he's made up in his head, without talking to Janelle. In fact, he realizes he has no idea what events or feelings might be preventing Janelle from calling him back.

But when he moves on to question 3, he discovers that when he believes that original thought, he's sad, he's angry, he's disappointed, and he's unwilling to reach out to Janelle and find out her side of the story.

And on question 4, when he considers who he would be without that thought, he finds a more patient, more compassionate James inside him, waiting to step forward.

Next, to deepen The Work still further, try flipping your original Judge Your Neighbor statement into a variety of opposite or inverted versions. In Katie's words, "This is an opportunity to experience the opposite of what you originally believed." It's especially powerful if you mentally experiment with ways that each of these statements *could* be true. When James plays with this, he writes these alternates:

- "I'm not calling Janelle back because I am mad at her after our conversation last week, and anyway I don't like her very much."
- "I am calling Janelle back because I like her very much, and appreciate her alternative perspectives."
- "For some reason, Janelle is not aware that I've been calling her."

- "For some reason, I am not aware that Janelle has been calling me back."
- Can you think of more ways that James could invert his original statement? Write them here:

_____

_____

_____

When James then asks the four "Is that true?" questions of each of these alternative frames, he learns more about what he knows and feels about himself, about Janelle, and even about phone calls and technology.

Try this exercise the next time you have an unpleasant thought about why someone is behaving toward you in a certain way, or why you feel you have to behave in a certain way toward them. Ask the 4 questions, and then try flipping the script in several ways, and asking the 4 questions of each of these new statements in turn.

Is Cynicism Toxic?

Life is certainly in the habit of pitching challenges to us, whether curve balls, screwballs or foul balls. When we are in burnout, our catcher's mitt is too often made in part of irritability and cynicism. In fact, as we discussed in Chapter 2, cynicism is a big part of the second dimension of burnout: Emotional Exhaustion, **Cynicism**, Inefficacy.

Nevertheless, cynicism can sometimes be a useful attitude. Let's find out when cynicism is helpful and when it is not, as well as some strategies for dealing with its unhelpful versions when they crop up.

A nicely succinct **definition of cynicism** is "a form of jaded negativity, and other times, realistic criticism or skepticism." That same definition goes on to mention:

- General distrust of others' apparent motives or ambitions
- Lack of faith or hope in the human race or in individuals
- Perceiving others' desires, hopes, opinions or personal tastes as unrealistic or inappropriate, therefore deserving of ridicule or admonishment

Regarding that part about "realistic criticism or skepticism," researchers say that **your occasional cynical moments can serve some useful roles in your life:**

- Cynicism and its cousin, satire, are valuable tools for situational criticism, which can lead to improved problem solving.
- When cynical statements also shock or surprise you, they may make you laugh. Laughter offers welcome relief from overwhelm.
- Cynicism is part of the capacity to feel suspicious of motives and bias — certainly useful in protecting yourself against gullibility.

In other words, a cynical moment may sometimes be a valuable Coping Skill. In that case, that bitter or suspicious feeling is warning you that you may have a problem that needs your attention. Once that unpleasant feeling has gotten your attention, the next step is to define the situation in a way that lets you handle it. You could decide it is absurd and laughable, or that it is a problem that needs solving, or that the feeling is warning you that deeper investigation into potential hidden motives or bias may be warranted.

However, **letting yourself get stuck in prolonged cynicism has big burnout downsides.** Research is increasingly suggesting that prolonged cynicism is associated with major health challenges. Research definitely shows that cynicism increases burnout's resemblance to that "workplace zombie virus" we discussed in Chapter 1, since cynical venting causes burnout to spread to others "like a contagion."

First, let's take a quick look at the **major health challenges associated with cynicism.**

Depression. When re-tested 19 years later, adults who had tested high in midlife on "cynical distrust" were 5 times more likely to experience depression, according to one large study.

Dementia. As we age, cynical distrust may be associated with an increased risk of developing dementia. Cynicism is a possible risk factor for dementia that is within our control to change.

Inflammation. Cynical distrust is also associated with an increase in three laboratory blood markers of systemic inflammation. The lab results of people who felt cynical distrust showed worse inflammation than people those for people who were stressed (who showed two markers) or depressed (who showed only one marker). It is true that researchers were not sure if it was the cynicism itself that caused the problem, or if cynical people tend to engage in more unhealthy behaviors (such as smoking or poor diet) that then cause inflammation. However, either way, decreasing cynicism will make your life better *now*.

Heart Disease. Cynicism seems to be associated with increased risk of cardiovascular diseases, such as heart attack and stroke.

Clearly, limiting our own cynical responses produces both possible health benefits and definite mood benefits.

Beth: Choosing Not to Vent

Recently, I walked into a meeting feeling tired, cranky, and annoyed at the failures of others. What's worse, my role that day was to provide a performance evaluation of the entire meeting, and highlight areas for improvement. Right from the beginning, I found plenty of failures upon which to unleash my annoyance.

The meeting started 10 minutes late. One of the principal contributors arrived even later. The AV tech issues had not been sorted out prior to the start of the meeting, leading to irritating delays. People who had committed to roles in the meeting had not shown up at all. A first-time visitor was being treated to a very poor impression of our work. To top it all off, I imagined that these failures meant that this group, which I deeply value and into which I have poured a lot of energy, might be in jeopardy of foundering, despite all of our best efforts.

My first impulse was to call the group to order on their many failures. I wanted to vent some thunder. "What are you thinking? You people know better! Straighten out!"

But I was uncomfortably aware that the burnout research is quite clear: venting is contagiously terrible in spreading burnout. Research also shows that the more positive statements made in a work session, the more productive the group will be. I knew I had to find a way to stand in front of this group and couch my message of accountability in positive terms. In short, I had to improve my Coping Skills style.

With all this in mind, I started listening with a different ear. In fact, once I started paying attention, I saw that everyone who had shown up that day, even—especially!—the guy who was late, were demonstrating too many strengths for me to cover, in the time allowed for my evaluation. I realized I would have to focus on the best.

When my time came, I opened with, "Despite the fact that we got off to a rough start, what I really appreciate is that everyone here stepped up. We had a lot of roles that had to be filled on the fly. No-one hesitated to volunteer, and everyone contributed beautifully." As I spoke on, I saw heads nodding, all over the room. Yes, they agreed with me: we certainly can do better. But they also agreed: look what we accomplished, despite it all!

Perhaps you are thinking: this is simply what any thoughtful leader would do: recognize performance strengths while demanding accountability. Indeed, you're right! Furthermore, I simply followed the guidelines of our group, which teaches that evaluations should be presented as a "sandwich:" that is, mention something good both before and after pointing out something that needs improvement.

The delightful discovery for me: my shift in focus improved the rest of my day. As I spoke, I was filled with no less than *love* for my whole team of professional colleagues. This feeling of love and appreciation buoyed me all through the rest of my long and busy day.

In burnout prevention terms: by choosing to notice and acknowledge the good in a stressful situation where I also needed to demand accountability, I was able to:

- Re-energize my own emotions,
- Re-connect with people I respect, and
- Do my part in building effectiveness in our group.

So much for burnout's three dimensions. Changing my Coping Skills style away from venting made my day.

Design a Vacation to Strengthen Your Burnout Shield

In Chapter1, we talked about burnout as a type of physical workplace injury. We challenge you to consider that when thinking about your next vacation, so that you set your primary purpose for your next vacation as *healing and recovery.*

Start by reviewing your vacation ideas and plans against your Burnout Shield. How well does your vacation plan support and foster your Self-Care, Reflection & Recognition, Capacity, Community and Coping Skills?

First, set a priority on your own Self-Care. Have a candid discussion about Self-Care priorities with those who will share your vacation, and compare your current definitions of "rest and relaxation." If you are exhausted, sleep may well be your overwhelming need, swamping all your other vacation plans (we mentioned a "Sleep Vacation" in Chapter 6.) Setting realistic expectations can head off frustration and disappointment.

Second, consider **what activities and scenery would nurture your Reflective mind,** your heart and soul.

- Do you need to turn quietly inward, for meditation or prayer? Or would you appreciate participating in a community that puts meditation or prayer at its center?
- Would immersion in natural beauty foster your ability for Reflection? If so, is your energy sufficient right now for hiking and camping, or would you be happier at this time staying in a room with a view, near a garden path?
- Are you someone who enjoys and draws inspiration from viewing great art? What sorts of art?
- Are you most Reflective when you have an opportunity to actively get involved in creative pursuits? Which arts or crafts? Again, would you appreciate participating in an arts or crafts community?
- Will humor help you recover your perspective? For you, would that mean hanging out with friends or family who make you laugh, attending comedy shows, or lining up a set of favorite funny movies to watch at home?

Third, **how strong is your functional Capacity** right now? And how much recovery time is available to you *after* your vacation is over? Would a high-exertion vacation nurture your Capacity right now?

Also, what is your financial Capacity? Setting a vacation budget that respects your current financial Capacity will help prevent having your vacation add to your stress.

Fourth, **in what ways can you strengthen your connections to your Community** while on vacation? Who would you love to spend time with? Do you need to make new friends or try out a new social group?

And fifth, **how will you bring your Coping Skills to bear on both the delights and challenges** a vacation creates? What Coping Skills will you need to muster to weather travel delays, lost luggage, miscommunications and so on? What Coping Skills will allow you to fully enjoy the moments and let the frustrations roll off your back?

Also, on your vacation, set your intention to stop *buzzing.* Buzzing is our word for being so busy that you forget how to stop: check email, do some tasks from the to-do list, check email, run errands, call people back, check email, pick up the kids, check email, grab a meal, check email…buzz, buzz, buzz. You may have to live with being a little bored, at first, until the pressure to keep buzzing lets up, and you can relax.

Did you know that you can enhance your enjoyment by developing your ability to savor life experiences? Set your intention to pack some of these **savoring skills** to bring with you on your vacation. (This list is modified from one in a terrific article on UC Berkeley's "Greater Good" website.)

- Share your good feelings with others.
- Take a mental photograph.
- Congratulate yourself.
- Sharpen your sensory perceptions — allow yourself to be highly attentive to what you see, hear and feel (avoid multitasking!)
- Express your good feelings in verbal and nonverbal ways.
- Compare the outcome to something worse.
- Let your attention get absorbed in the moment.
- Count your blessings and give thanks.
- Avoid killjoy thinking.
- Remind yourself how quickly time flies.

Expect the Right Beach

On a recent hot summer day, two women friends loaded their tall standard poodle into the car and drove to the Oregon coast. It was a beautiful Pacific Northwest morning at the beach. The air was a refreshing 20 degrees cooler than inland, the fog was just starting to recede, and the steel gray ocean was rolling beautiful white-topped waves shoreward, past the silhouetted Haystack rock.

As they laughingly threw the ball for the dog (who was highly indignant that the ball kept getting *sand* on it,) a young man approached them. "I'm visiting from Cuba," he said, as he shook their hands. Then he leaned in close to one of them and whispered, as politely as he could, "What is wrong with this beach? It's really ugly!"

It turned out, the poor guy had been expecting a Caribbean beach! His expectations kept him from enjoying the cool soft muted tones of the beach he was on.

When you plan your time off, set your expectations for the events you'll actually be experiencing (which may include a *lot* of sleeping in.) If you are expecting a Caribbean vacation when this trip is in the Pacific Northwest vacation, then you will be disappointed, like that young Cuban man. Why not "expect the right beach" from the beginning?

Using Humor

Humor is such a valuable coping tool. It is one of the rare skills that can be useful as both a problem-focused and an emotion-focused skill. It can help you approach people, open discussion on sensitive topics, bond people together, make light of an otherwise bleak situation, and it usually feels good for everyone involved.

In short, when you use humor, try to follow a few basic guidelines: stay away from humor that is hurtful in nature or made at someone else's (or your organization's) expense. Otherwise, humor can be a valuable tool in your collection of coping skills.

If you don't feel comfortable using humor at work, you can try a couple different strategies to bring humor more into your life. First, make a point to laugh or acknowledge other people who use humor around you. Second, seek out humorous entertainment that is related to your type of situation. If you are feeling stressed or overwhelmed, laughter really can be some of the best medicine.

Below, we share a great humorous essay by Tara Rolstad, whom you met earlier in this chapter. It illustrates some reframing, too. Enjoy!

Celebrate Your Best Bad

By Tara Rolstad

Grilled cheese, singing, playing poker, loading furniture in car, remembering I'm lactose intolerant. All things I'm bad at. They're my bad. What about you, what's your bad?

But wait, there's more.

I'm a bad driver. I'm a bad manager. I'm a bad stay-at-home mom. Who admits that? These are all things I've said and believed about myself.

Today, I share with you three questions to help you break down the self-limiting statement "I'm bad at that," and understand it. Then forget all of this societal peer pressure to "be your best." You can celebrate your bad!

Why not? I mean, used to be, you pretty much had to be or live with a farmer, a laborer, builder, a tailor or seamstress, a tool crafter, a roofer, a plumber, EWWW drains??? I can't do any of that, and it's OK. We don't HAVE to good at everything anymore.

But...Socrates said, "An unexamined life is not worth living." I would argue that the same is true for unexamined bad, which is not worth...badding....Well, I haven't fully fleshed out the comparative metaphor but I feel strongly about it. If you don't examine your bad, you risk:

- Missing out on adventure.
- Missing out on a deeper understanding of who you are, and who you are capable of being, and allowing us to miss out too.
- Missing out on burning calories. Being bad means failure, and Failure burns fat. Check the Interwebs, people, that's science right there.

So here are the three questions to ask yourself:

Does your bad have an upside?

I'm not talking a cheesy "I'm too much of a perfectionist," or "I intimidate people with my perfection" but what is the REAL value in your bad. *What does your bad bring to the table?*

Take grilled cheese—I can't make a grilled cheese sandwich to save my life. Burnt, crunchy, smoky and bad, every time. So on grilled cheese and tomato soup night at my house, my children have the blessing of seeing their dad as a competent and nurturing provider in the kitchen, and I get to eat grilled cheese. Not only that, but it made me mad I couldn't master such a simple skill. So I dug in, did more research, and I discovered the secret to the grilled cheese sandwich. (The secret to a great grilled cheese? It's mayonnaise. You're welcome.)

Are you really globally bad, or is your definition of the role or activity too limited?

Sometimes we allow ourselves to believe that because we do not reach the general definition of good than we are bad, when in fact we are merely bad at parts of the role; maybe parts that don't even matter to us, and we rock at parts of the role for which we are uniquely gifted. We've got to break it down.

I'm a bad driver. No I'm not, I'm a bad parker...and un-parker. *"Public service announcement for the audience, tonight's speaker is currently driving a blue Toyota Prius. Please use caution when exiting the parking lot."*

I'm a bad manager. No, I'm not, I'm great at building teams, making the work fun, and enrolling people to a cause! I'm bad at minor little parts of the role that don't interest or excite me. You know, budgets, spreadsheets, timelines, budget-y things...

But what do we lose when we just accept we are bad at something? What if I have an amazing hidden talent at plumbing? Let's be clear, I'm still not gonna do it, 'cause gross.

But...what if you have the potential to be a life-changing translator of ancient Gaelic poetry, but you gave up on languages in the ninth grade when your Spanish teacher spent all of the class lecturing you on the nuanced details of Sandinistan politics and teaching you curse words? Maybe you're not bad at languages, you're just bad at caring about Central American politics, or you are too shy to ever use the good swear words! *(Too specific of an example? I can't imagine why...)*

For me the most difficult was saying and believing **I was a bad stay-at-home mom.** But I'm not good at preschool crafts. I could not get trips to the park right; apparently they needed snacks, sunscreen, diapers, EVERY TIME; and every time it was a surprise to me. I wasn't a Pinterest mom, I didn't color coordinate or decorate or blah-blah-ate. Most of all, the house was, and is, always a mess. So I believed it, believed I was a bad stay-at-home mom.

That's just a recipe for poor self-esteem and worse coping skills!

Until I realized I was great with frogs and snakes and laser tag and rocks and adventures and road trips; I realized I was a GREAT mom. I may be bad at crafts, I'm not Pinterest-y, and I'm a bad housekeeper. I can live with that!

What if you are really objectively bad? Do you, in fact, suck? That brings me to the final question. **If you really suck, you**

must ask yourself: does it still bring you joy? If it does, then you must find a way to do it anyways!

I'm a terrible singer. Awful. But I enjoy it, and so I sing. Unless it's a small Happy Birthday ensemble, then I lip sync.

Don't accept your bad. Understand it, define it, and then celebrate your best bad!

(Cue the song in your head, go on now. "Celebrate your bad, come on!")

Chapter ELEVEN

Staying Out of Burnout

"Resilience is how you recharge, not how you endure."
—*Shawn Achor*

How Will You Stay Vigilant Against Burnout?

Thank you for taking this journey with us! After working your way through this book, we hope you have a clearer understanding of what is critical not only to your productivity, but also to your energy and to your full enjoyment of your life.

When you are a hard worker, it is easy to give up things in order to prioritize whatever you have deemed is "most important." Sometimes, in the short term, it can be necessary to do so. But when such pressured activity becomes the norm again for you, then you risk burnout creeping back into your life.

Use the exercises in this chapter to help you prepare for those times. Good risk management is a cycle: *identify* the problems, *evaluate* solutions, *mitigate* the problems using the solutions you chose, and *monitor* progress.

With just a little prep up front (identify and evaluate), you'll be ready to shoo away the burnout beast (mitigate) whenever it attempts to show its head in your life again (monitor). Here are the details on these action-oriented steps you can take to ready your burnout risk management plan.

Interactive: Identify—Your Vital Burnout Protection Info

1. Your **personal warning signs.** What behaviors pop up for you, when you are feeling overwhelmed, overstressed, or burned out? Examples: cursing at traffic, snapping at co-workers or family members, increase in minor injuries...(You may have already made your list in Chapter 3. If so, feel free to copy it here):

_____

_____

_____

2. Looking back, what were important **factors in your environment that led to your previous burnout?** These are triggers to watch out for, if they recur (or are still present). For this list, we'll rely first on Maslach and Leiter's *6 areas of worklife* (and then add in some other factors, too.) These two important burnout researchers found that you are at a much higher risk of burnout when mismatches occur between your work environment and your own needs in any of these six areas.

Make a brief note if any of these factors played a role in burnout for you:

_____

_____

_____

Workload: When workload was a mismatch for you, there was consistently too much to do, too little time, too few resources. After especially demanding stretches, your opportunities to recover may also have been inadequate.

_____

_____

_____

Control: Control mismatch existed when you generally did not have the feeling of being able to influence decisions that affect your work, were not able to exercise professional autonomy or did not have access to the resources necessary to do an effective job. Control mismatch also includes **role conflict**, defined as a mismatch between what you enjoy or what you're good at, on the one hand, and what your work had you doing, on the other.

_____

_____

_____

Reward: Reward mismatch means monetary compensation, social connections and recognition, or work pleasure and satisfaction were not consistent with your expectations.

_____

_____

_____

Community: Community mismatch may have occurred for you, if the overall quality of social interaction at work was poor, including issues of conflict, mutual support, closeness, and the capacity to work as a team. Did you experience trust, humor, respect...?

_____

_____

Fairness: A fairness mismatch existed when you did not perceive the decisions at work as fair and you felt people are not treated with respect.

Values: Was there conflict between your personal ideals and motivations which originally attracted you to this work, and the values of the organization?

Beyond Maslach and Leiter's 6 worklife areas, studies suggest other stressors also have a strong impact on your burnout risk. Make a note here if any of these other factors helped lead to your previous burnout:

Health challenges (your own or your family's):

Financial stressors:

_____

_____

_____

Interpersonal stressors (if you need to, refer to the Holmes and Rahe scale in Chapter 5):

_____

_____

_____

Internal factors. These would have become a burnout issue if there was a mismatch between your personality style and your work environment. Examples include: Where you sit on the introversion/extroversion continuum when compared with your opportunities to be social in groups. Another is your tendency to be mainly promotion-focused or prevention-focused when compared with the use by those around you of goal-setting approaches or problem-solving approaches.

_____

_____

_____

Interactive: Evaluate—What Works For You

1. **Stress forecasting:** You can often predict some future times when you might need to step up the burnout prevention because you may be more vulnerable to stress. Let's take a look.

Sun	Mon	Tue	Wed	Thu	Fri
			1	2	3
3	4	7	8	9	10
10	11	14	15	16	17
17	18		22	23	24
24	25			30	
31					

Times of year that are more stressful for you than others (holidays, production calendars, fiscal year end, etc.):

_____

_____

_____

Potential life or personal events that tend to increase your stress level, distract your efforts, or otherwise decrease your ability to deal with stress:

_____

_____

_____

Your support team. List at least three positive, trustworthy people you can call on when you need help or a different perspective:

Whom do you admire for their healthy response to stress?

_____

_____

_____

Who do you know has good intentions toward you?

_____

_____

_____

Is there someone who might actually be upset if you *didn't* ask them for help when you were really in need?

_____

_____

_____

2. **What is meaningful for you?** What do you live for? What do you work for?

_____

_____

_____

Daily reflection cues. Also note what sensory cues remind you to take a few minutes for reflection. Fill in at least 2 items that work for you:

Time of day: _____

Reminder on daily calendar or task list _____

Sensory cues: What do I see, hear, smell (coffee?) or how I feel:

_____

_____

3. In your five Burnout Shield Key Areas, list the **changes** you've made that have, so far, **made the biggest difference for you** in each area:

Self-Care

_____

_____

_____

Reflection & Recognition

_____

_____

_____

Capacity

_____

_____

Community

_____

_____

_____

Coping Styles

_____

_____

_____

Interactive: Mitigate & Monitor—Your Burnout First Aid Action Plan

Yikes! How do you manage a High Burnout Risk Alert? Here is how you use the information you collected above to manage a High Stress Burnout Alert in your life.

If you notice one of your stress warning signs: STOP!

Step 1. Pause what you are doing (when it is safe to do so).

Step 2. Identify any additional warning signs. Do you need immediate care?

_____

_____

_____

Step 3. Do a quick mental review of your Burnout Shield. How are you doing in the five areas of vulnerability: Self-Care, Reflection & Recognition, Capacity, Community and Coping Skills? Have you recently stopped doing something that had been protecting you? Anything you need to add?

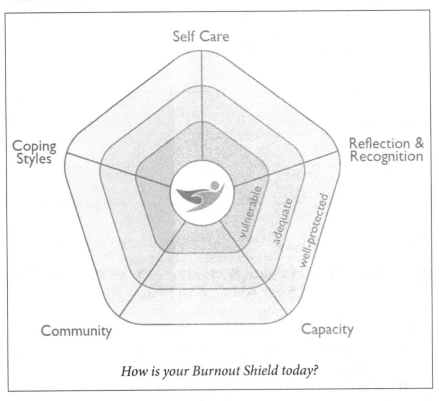

How is your Burnout Shield today?

Step 4: If there are new stressors or mismatch factors in your life, are they short-term or long-term? Do you have control over any of these new changes that make you more vulnerable to burnout?

Step 5: Considering the short-term or long-term nature of your stressors, identify what you can do to increase your protection or decrease risk against burnout.

In other words, if you feel the straw's about to break the camel's back, how can you lighten the load? Here's a reminder of some of the quick suggestions that appeared in Chapters 6 through 10, for each of the five Key Areas of your Burnout Shield.

Self-Care. Are you taking care of yourself and providing the basic things that keep your body going? Do some of these basics as soon as possible:

Take 10 slow deep breaths.

Drink some water.

Eat some nourishing food.

Take a bathroom break.

Get some rest.

Reflection & Recognition. This comprises two sections.

Reflect now. Name at least one meaningful thing that happened today.

_____

_____

Recognize yourself now. Name your own accomplishments today, including the smaller ones and the interim steps you've taken toward larger achievements.

_____

_____

Capacity. Are you aware of how much you can take and how close you are to that limit? What can you Delay, Delegate or Drop?

_____

_____

Community. Look back at your list above, of who you can ask for help, delegate work to, ask for guidance or gain perspective from. Are you getting the social interaction you need? What community would or does make you welcome?

_____

_____

Coping Skills. Review the flow chart at the beginning of Chapter Ten. What coping style might better serve you, today?

_____

_____

Step 6: You've just created your plan! Carry it out. Remember to start small, be gentle with yourself, and recognize your accomplishments along the way.

Step 7: Monitor: Set a time to check in with yourself again.

Step 8: Repeat this process as needed.

Keep In Mind…

We created this book in the hope that your journey out of burnout would be less bumpy than ours. Along the way, we've shared many precepts that for us were hard won. Please keep these essential points in mind:

You Are Not Alone

While burnout is certainly not the result of a workplace zombie virus, it is at epidemic levels. If you've been suffering through burnout, we suspect that some of your colleagues are, as well. If you've found this book helpful, please share it with them.

Burnout Is Physical

We see burnout as a kind of repetitive stress injury. To review from Chapter 1, we identified these ways in which burnout is similar to other types of injuries:

- Your performance and overall capacity are affected.
- Recovery requires a healing process.
- This healing process takes time.
- Rest is a necessary component of recovery.
- Some of your daily habits will need to change as you recover.
- Specific exercises will help rebuild your strength and resiliency.
- If you continue as if you aren't injured, you could hurt yourself even more.
- Telling the difference between helpful and hurtful activities isn't necessarily common sense.
- Nobody feels like they have time to be injured; injuries are seldom convenient.
- The best way to get better is to take the healing process seriously and commit to it.
- You will not be like this forever, you can recover.

Burnout Is Also Mental, Emotional and Spiritual

Burnout's triad of exhaustion, disconnection, and lack of purpose can feel like a whole set of different problems. Don't let this variety of issues fool you as to the underlying cause: burnout. Use your Burnout Shield to help you recover, and *get help now* if you are in great distress.

Please, please, be gentle with yourself as you recover. Because burnout is so misunderstood in the modern world, it can be easy to believe burnout is the result of weakness or inadequacy. The truth is, you are a rock star. And rock stars that last are the ones that build regular recharging into their lives.

Your Burnout May Look Different

In Chapter 4 we discussed the three main types of burnout:
- Frenetic
- Worn-out
- Underchallenged (*aka* "Boreout" — so bored you're burned out)

There Is Plenty of Hope

There are certainly a lot of "external" causes of burnout, as you noted in the first worksheet in this chapter, and many of them may be outside your control. However, if your external environment is not likely to change for the better (and even if it is) there is still plenty you can personally do about it, in five Key Areas, using your Burnout Shield. Your situation is full of hope.

If you haven't yet done so, please go back now and do the Burnout Shield Self-Tests in Chapter 5.

Remember to Recharge

Get the five areas of the Burnout Shield into your head. Whether you visualize it as a knight's buckler blocking whatever is coming at you, or a futuristic force field that surrounds and protects you on every side (or you have some other mental picture that works for you), the Burnout Shield can serve as your go-to reference for a quick check-in on how you're keeping burnout at bay, so you can survive and thrive.

We built the Burnout Shield to be much more than a random collection of tips. It is your KISSY system: **K**eep **I**t **S**imple, **S**ave **Y**ourself. By reviewing your Burnout Shield, you can quickly use it as a source of information for something new to add, when you are ready for more ways to recharge your energy and productivity.

Our clients have discovered a number of other ways to make use of the system. They suggest you take a mental glance over your Burnout Shield dashboard when:

Your "rumble strip" **personal warning signs** show up in your life, as described in the first section of this chapter.

When you're **considering dropping a pleasurable activity** out of your life. Do the Burnout Shield benefits of this activity outweigh the areas where it stresses your Shield? If so, you might consider putting that activity back in your life as soon as you possibly can.

You are "speeding," or even **tempted to overstretch yourself** again. In fact, if you're considering any new project or commitment, take it through a quick mental whirl around your Burnout Shield, asking the same question as above: Do the Burnout Shield benefits of this activity outweigh the areas where it stresses your Shield? If they do not, and you still want to take it on, your next question to ask your Shield: what can I do to protect my Capacity?

You feel you are **running out of gas**. When your energy or interest flags, that's another good time to do a quick mental review of your Shield. What strategy would help, right now? We both do this, every day. With our go-getter attitudes, we really need these reminders to help us "walk our talk!'"

You are **"driving" well.** As any good driver does, teach yourself to glance frequently at your dashboard once a day or so. In any of the five Key Areas, is the internal meter beginning to drift toward the red zone? Prevention is *so* much easier than cure!

You want to **teach good "driving"** to others. In our experience working with a wide variety of clients, the Burnout Shield dashboard is useful for people in many professions and different life situations. If it has helped you, please do pass it along!

Tell us How You Are Doing!

We would love to hear from you. Join our community! You can communicate with us directly via the Burnout Solutions Facebook page: follow us, and post your comments and questions at https://www.facebook.com/burnoutsolutions/. Please share what is working for you, so that the whole community will benefit. On that page you can also learn new ideas — we frequently share new up-to-date resources.

If you prefer to email us, hop over to http://www.burnout-solutions.com/contact/. We'll get right back to you.

You Matter

Burnout is not a badge of honor or of shame. It's a consequence of unrelieved stress. Regardless of whether your environment is subject to change, you can recover. We did it, you can do it too.

From our hearts to yours: Your work matters. Your health matters. Your values matter. Your family and community matter. Learn to value yourself, your health and your stamina. We care about you and need you. Your friends, your family and your community need you.

Nurture yourself, because **you matter.**

Appendices

Appendix A

Recommended Reading

Here are some books, articles and videos we like very much, and which have affected our understanding of burnout and recovery. For those topics most interesting to you, they would provide fascinating additional information.

Achor, S. (2010). *The happiness advantage: the seven principles of positive psychology that fuel success and performance at work*. New York: Broadway Books.

Ariga, A., & Lleras, A. (2011). Brief and rare mental "breaks" keep you focused: Deactivation and reactivation of task goals preempt vigilance decrements. *Cognition, 118*(3), 439–443. doi:10.1016/j.cognition.2010.12.007

Blanchard, K. H., Oncken, W., & Burrows, H. (1989). *The one minute manager meets the monkey*. New York: Morrow.

Bolles, R. N. (2017). *What color is your parachute?: a practical manual for job-hunters and career-changers*. Berkeley: Ten Speed Press.

Crowley, C., & Lodge, H. S. (2004). *Younger next year: a guide to living like 50 until you're 80 and beyond*. New York: Workman Pub.

T. (2012, December 05). Forget big change, start with a tiny habit: BJ Fogg at TEDxFremont. Retrieved February 02, 2017, from http://www.youtube.com/watch?v=AdKUJxjn-R8

Friedman, R. (2014, November 05). Schedule a 15-minute break before you burn out. Retrieved February 02, 2017, from https://hbr.org/2014/08/schedule-a-15-minute-break-before-you-burn-out

I'm Fine, Thanks: A Documentary. (n.d.). Retrieved February 22, 2017, from http://www.imfinethanksmovie.com/. Directed by Grant Peele.

Jarka, R., PhD. (2014, October 31). The Miracle Minute. Retrieved February 23, 2017, from https://www.youtube.com/watch?v=if2ptQz7YP4

Kabat-Zinn, J. (1991). *Full catastrophe living: using the wisdom of your body and mind to face stress, pain, and illness.* New York, NY: Pub. by Dell Pub., a division of Bantam Doubleday Dell Pub. Group.

Lyubomirsky, S. (2008). *The how of happiness: a scientific approach to getting the life you want.* New York: Penguin Press.

McGonigal, J. (2010, February). Gaming can make a better world. Retrieved February 02, 2017, from https://www.ted.com/talks/jane_mcgonigal_gaming_can_make_a_better_world

Rath, T. (2007). *Strengths finder 2.0.* New York: Gallup.

Appendix B

Game-based Interactive Learning: A Process of Elimination

As we said in Chapter Six, you can learn lots of great stuff when it comes to healthy personal habits. To make this topic a lot more fun, try this Quiz.

Answer these trivia questions and then check the explanations as you read through the answer key. Enjoy!

1. How much water should you drink in a day?
A. Enough to keep you from feeling thirsty
B. Enough so you urinate every two to 4 hours, and your urine is light yellow
C. Sixty 8-ounce glasses every day
D. A+B
E. B+C

_____

2. How can you get more bathroom breaks?
A. Set a timer for every 2 hours. (Don't ignore it!)
B. Build a team who can cover your responsibilities when necessary. Someone on the team will watch your patients or your students until you get back from the restroom, and you do the same for some of them.
C. Avoid multitasking
D. All of the above

_____

3. What percentage of US adults eat the recommended amounts of fiber daily (38 g/day for men, 25 g/day for women)?

A. Less than 3%
B. Less than 5%
C. About 30%
D. 45%
E. The majority   _____

4. Which of the following are good sources of fiber?

A. Steak
B. Red beans and rice
C. Hummus
D. Apples
E. Cranberry juice
F. Whole plants
G. B, C, D, and F   _____

5. Which has *more fiber?*

One pear or 1/2 cup of dried prunes.

A. Pear
B. Prunes
C. Equal to each other   _____

One persimmon or 1/2 cup of dried figs.

D. Persimmon
E. Figs
F. Equal to each other   _____

Half an avocado or one banana.

G. Avocado
H. Banana
I. Equal to each other   _____

Sunflower seeds or almonds.

J. Sunflower seeds
K. Almonds
L. Equal to each other   _____

Spinach or Swiss chard.

M. Spinach
N. Chard
O. Equal to each other   _____

Medium sweet potato with skin, or medium russet (brown) potato with skin.

P. Sweet
Q. Russet
R. Equal to each other   _____

Raspberries or blueberries.

S. Raspberries
T. Blueberries
U. Equal to each other   _____

6. Which are benefits of eating more fiber and drinking more water?

A. Helps control blood sugar (by decreasing highs and lows)
B. Assists weight loss
C. Lowers cholesterol
D. Encourages the growth of beneficial bacteria in your gut
E. Reduces the calorie density of foods
F. All of the above
G. None of the above   _____

Answers to A Process of Elimination

1. D is correct. The combination of answers A+B is correct. In 2004, the Institute of Medicine of the National Academy reviewed years of research evidence on adequate water intake and has the following recommendations: (Note: a "cup" is equivalent to an 8-ounce glass; they assume that some of your fluid intake comes from foods like fruits and vegetables, which have a high water content.)

Men: 13 cups (about 10.5 cups from beverages)

Women: 9 cups (about 7 cups from beverages)

Pregnant women: 10 cups (about 8 cups from beverages)

Breastfeeding women: 13 cups (about 10.5 cups from beverages)

Add more water if you are physically active or in a hot climate.

A. Yes, but while important, avoiding thirst is not enough. Thirst occurs late in dehydration. Mild thirst is also too easy to ignore.

B. Yes. Your urine should be light yellow, but not pale yellow. Note: "Urine color doesn't work for everyone. Taking dietary supplements that contain riboflavin will make your urine bright yellow, and certain medications can change the color of your urine, as well. And if you have any kidney problems or other heath conditions you should talk to your health care provider about how much water to drink."

C. Nope. 60 glasses would be terribly too much for you to drink. Drinking that much in a day would cause some severe health problems.

2. D. Actually, any or all of the answers are correct. All three strategies can help you take the bathroom breaks you need.

A. The timer alarm can create a great excuse: "Oh! Excuse me, I have an appointment."

B. Some colleagues and some administrators can create a discouraging atmosphere around breaks. To counter this, center your pitch for respecting break time on three things:

- Improved productivity comes from opportunities to rest and refresh
- Breaks decrease costly or dangerous errors that might otherwise occur due to dehydration and discomfort
- Morale improves when teams support each other

C. Multitasking decreases your ability to pay enough attention to any of the things you're doing, let alone tune in to your own biological signals. Avoiding multitasking helps you take breaks when you need to.

3. A is correct.

The Institute of Medicine recommends dietary fiber intake for adults up to age 50 of 38 grams for men and 25 grams for women; for men and women older than 50, an intake of 30 and 21 grams, respectively. But Americans have an actual average intake of about 15 grams per day. Another way to think about this: Consume 14 grams of fiber for every 1000 calories you eat. So if you eat 2000 calories per day, you should also be getting 28 grams of fiber. Some nutrition authorities think even these recommended numbers for daily fiber intake are too low. They recommend you eat foods containing a total of 40–50 grams per day of fiber.

4. G. is correct.

A. Nope. No meat has dietary fiber. Don't confuse dietary fiber with foods that have a "fibrous" mouth feel.

B. Yes. All beans are terrific sources of fiber. A cup of cooked black beans or pinto beans has 15 grams of fiber; while Whole grain rice, such as brown rice, with 4 grams of fiber, is a much better source of fiber than white rice, which only has 0.6 grams of fiber.

C. Yes. Hummus — and any other food made with lots of chickpeas — is a great source of fiber, with each tablespoon supplying about 1 gram of fiber. (Some versions of hummus may come with a high load of added oil and salt, however.)

D. Yes. Apples have lots of lovely fiber, about 4 grams. (Be sure to eat the peel, too.)

E. Nope. Not cranberry juice. When you drink just the juice of any fruit (or veggie), you lose out on its fiber.

F. Yes. Plants! All whole plant foods contain fiber.

5. Which has more fiber?

C: **Equal**. Either 1 medium pear or 1/2 cup of dried prunes gives you 6 grams of fiber.

E: Figs. The dried figs add up to 8 grams of fiber, while the persimmon gives you 6 grams.

G. Avocado. Half an avocado gives you 9 grams of fiber, while a medium banana gives you only 3 grams.

K. Almonds. An ounce of almonds has 4 grams of fiber, while an ounce of sunflower seeds has about 3 grams.

O. Equal. A cup of either spinach or Swiss chard, cooked, yields 4 grams of fiber.

R. Equal. Either potato, a medium russet or medium sweet, with skin, yields 4 grams of fiber.

S. Raspberries. 1 cup of raspberries gives you 8 grams of fiber; the same amount of blueberries give you 4 grams of fiber.

Note: Every one of the foods listed under question 5 is a great nutritional choice. Each gives you lots of other nutritional benefits, in addition to their fiber content.

6. F. All the benefits listed in this question are true benefits of eating whole foods in a fiber-rich diet and drinking more water.

For more information about common food sources and their levels of dietary fiber, check out health.gov and the dietary guideline resources available there, including a chart of *Food Sources of Dietary Fiber.*

A Process of Elimination, What Now?

So — how did you do on this mini-quiz? What did you learn?

Did any of this information surprise you?

If you discovered you need to make some changes, write ONE thing you are going to change this week:

Appendix C

Sources and References

Many of these reference materials served as sources for more than one of the chapters in this book. Since this list, as printed, is already quite long, we did not repeat the citation for each chapter in which the ideas appear.

Sources for Chapter ONE: Contrary to Popular Belief, Burnout is Not a Workplace Zombie Virus

Ahola, K., Salminen, S., Toppinen-Tanner, S., Koskinen, A., & Väänänen, A. (2013). Occupational burnout and severe injuries: An eight-year prospective cohort study among Finnish forest industry workers. *Journal of Occupational Health, 55*(6), 450–457. doi:10.1539/joh.13-0021-oa

Cimiotti, J. P., Aiken, L. H., Sloane, D. M., & Wu, E. S. (2012). Nurse staffing, burnout, and health care–associated infection. *American Journal of Infection Control, 40*(6), 486–490. doi:10.1016/j.ajic.2012.02.029

DiCarlo, M., & Albert Shanker Institute. (2015, January 22). Update on teacher turnover in the U.S. Retrieved February 08, 2017, from http://www.shankerinstitute.org/blog/update-teacher-turnover-us

Embriaco, N., Azoulay, E., Barrau, K., Kentish, N., Pochard, F., Loundou, A., & Papazian, L. (2007). High level of burnout in intensivists. *American Journal of Respiratory and Critical Care Medicine, 175*(7), 686–692. doi:10.1164/rccm.200608-1184oc

Enoch, L., Chibnall, J. T., Schindler, D. L., & Slavin, S. J. (2013). Association of medical student burnout with residency specialty choice. *Medical Education, 47*(2), 173–181. doi:10.1111/medu.12083

Hassard, Juliet, and Małgorzata Milczarek. *Calculating the cost of work-related stress and psychosocial risks literature review.* Bilbao:

The European Agency for Safety and Health at Work (EU-OSHA), 2014. Print. Appendix III: Cost Indicators for psychological disorders in the workplace (Brun and Lamarche, 2006)

Ingersoll, R., Merrill, L., & Stuckey, D. (2014). *Seven trends: the transformation of the teaching force, updated April 2014* (Rep. No. CPRE Report #RR-80). Philadelphia, PA: Consortium for Policy Research in Education, University of Pennsylvania.

Jean Wallace discusses the importance of physician wellness [Audio blog interview: Lancet Podcast]. (2009, November 13). Retrieved from http://www.thelancet.com/journals/lancet/article/PIIS0140-6736(09)61424-0/abstract

Jones, C. B. (2008). Revisiting nurse turnover costs. *JONA: The Journal of Nursing Administration, 38*(1), 11–18. doi:10.1097/01.nna.0000295636.03216.6f

Kelly, G. (2015, April 29). 12 Telling points about physician stress and burnout. Retrieved May 04, 2017, from http://www.mdmag.com/physicians-money-digest/columns/the-doctor-report/04-2015/12-Telling-Points-About-Physician-Stress-and-Burnout

Legassie, J., Zibrowski, E. M., & Goldszmidt, M. A. (2008). Measuring resident well-being: Impostorism and burnout syndrome in residency. *journal of General Internal Medicine, 23*(7), 1090–1094. doi:10.1007/s11606-008-0536-x

Linzer, M., Visser, M. R., Oort, F. J., Smets, E. M., McMurray, J. E., & Haes, H. C. (2001). Predicting and preventing physician burnout: results from the United States and the Netherlands. *The American Journal of Medicine, 111*(2), 170–175. doi:10.1016/s0002-9343(01)00814-2

Meltzer-Brody, S., MD. (2014, July 2). Physician burnout: it's time to take care of our own. Retrieved October 4, 2015, from http://thehealthcareblog.com/blog/2014/07/02/physician-burnout-its-time-to-take-care-of-our-own/

Phillips, O., & NPR. (2015, March 30). Revolving door of teachers costs schools billions every year. Retrieved February 08, 2017, from http://www.npr.org/sections/ed/2015/03/30/395322012/the-hidden-costs-of-teacher-turnover

Rentner, D. S., Kober, N., Frizzell, M., Ferguson, M., Aigner, B., & Center on Education Policy. (2016, May). Listen to us: teacher views and voices. Retrieved February 08, 2017, from http://www.csai-online.org/resources/listen-us-teacher-views-and-voices

Shanafelt, T. D., Bradley, K. A., Wipf, J. E., & Back, A. L. (2002). Burnout and self-reported patient care in an internal medicine residency program. *Annals of Internal Medicine, 136*(5), 358. doi:10.732 6/0003-4819-136-5-200203050-00008

Shanafelt, T. D., Boone, S., Tan, L., Dyrbye, L. N., Sotile, W., Satele, D. . . . Oreskovich, M. R. (2012). Burnout and satisfaction with work-life balance among US physicians relative to the general US population. *Archives of Internal Medicine, 172*(18), 1377. doi:10.1001/archinternmed.2012.3199

Slavin, S. J., & Chibnall, J. T. (2016). Finding the why, changing the how. *Academic Medicine, 91*(9), 1194–1196. doi:10.1097/acm. 0000000000001226

Sources for Statistics in "Who Is At Risk for Burnout?"

Buick, I., and Thomas, M. (2001) "Why do middle managers in hotels burn out?" *International Journal of Contemporary Hospitality Management*, Vol. 13 No: 6, pp.304 – 309. DOI http://dx.doi.org/10.1108/EUM0000000005968

CareerBuilder Survey press release, (2013) More than one third of employed health care workers plan to look for a new job this year, CareerBuilder health care study reveals. Accessed at: http://www.careerbuilder.com/share/aboutus/pressreleasesdetail.aspx?sd=4%2F3 0%2F2013&id=pr754&ed=12%2F31%2F2013

Cook, S. (2015). Job burnout of information technology workers, *International Journal of Business, Humanities and Technology* Vol. 5, No. 3; June 2015

Doolittle, Benjamin R. (2007). Burnout and coping among parish-based clergy. *Mental Health, Religion & Culture*, Volume 10, Issue 1, pp 31–38. doi: 10.1080/13674670600857591

EFC, Efinancial Careers, authors not given, (2014). Career satisfaction and retention. Finance professionals in 2014: Career driven, loyalists or opportunists? Accessed at http://news-cdn.efinancialcareers.com/wp-content/uploads/2014/06/eFC-ENG-Retention-WP-JUN2014-sm.pdf?_ga=1.238224256.1627406752.1466518934

Farber, Barry A. (1991), Crisis in education: Stress and burnout in the American teacher. The Jossey-Bass education series. San Francisco, CA, US: Jossey-Bass Crisis in education: Stress and burnout in the American teacher. XXI 351 pp.

Francis, L., Wulff, K., & Robbins, M. (2008). The relationship between work-related psychological health and psychological type among clergy serving in the Presbyterian Church (USA). *Journal of Empirical Theology*, 21, 166–182. doi:10.1163/157092508X349854.

Harrison, S. and Gordon, P.A. (2014). Misconceptions of employee turnover: Evidence-based information for the retail grocery industry. *Journal of Business & Economics Research*, Second Quarter 2014 Volume 12, Number 2

Ingersoll, R. M. (2001). Teacher turnover and teacher shortages: an organizational analysis. *American Educational Research Journal*, 38(3), 499–534. doi:10.3102/00028312038003499

Kowalski, K.M.and Podlesny, A. (2002). The effects of disaster on workers: A study of burnout in investigators of serious accidents and fatalities in the U.S. mining industry. *Int J Emergency Management*, Vol 1, No 2.; 155–169

McCarty, W. P., Schuck, A., Skogan, W., and Rosenbaum, D. (2011). Stress, burnout, and health. Report from National Police Research Platform, funded by National Institute of Justice, accessed at http://static1.1.sqspcdn.com/static/f/733761/10444483/1296183365827/Stress+Burnout++and+Health+FINAL.pdf?token=2WfkiM2B2wNKM31xHV4xNn1LEjo%3D

MacDonald, J. B., Saliba, A. J., Hodgins, G., & Ovington, L. A. (2016). Burnout in journalists: A systematic literature review. *Burnout Research*, 3(2), 34–44. doi:10.1016/j.burn.2016.03.001

McHugh MD, Kutney-Lee A, Cimiotti JP, Sloane DM, Aiken LH. Nurses' widespread job dissatisfaction, burnout, and frustration with health benefits signal problems for patient care. *Health Aff (Millwood)*. 2011; 30(2):202–210.

Morse, G., Salyers, M. P., Rollins, A. L., Monroe-DeVita, M., and Pfahler, C. (2012) Burnout in mental health services: a review of the problem and its remediation. *Adm Policy Ment Health*. 2012 September; 39(5): 341–352. doi:10.1007/s10488-011-0352-1

Peckham, C. (2015). Physician burnout: It just keeps getting worse. *Medscape Family Medicine*, accessed at http://www.medscape.com/viewarticle/838437.

Reinardy, S. (2011). Newspaper journalism in crisis: Burnout on the rise, eroding young journalists' career commitment. *Journalism*, Vol. 12 no. 1, pp 33–50

Shani, Amir and Pizam, Abraham (2009). Work-related depression among hotel employees , *Cornell Hospitality Quarterly, OnlineFirst,* September 2, 2009 as DOI: 10.1177/1938965509344294

Staples Advantage Workplace Index 2016; http://www.staplesadvantage. com/sites/workplace-index/

Virginia, S. G. (1998); Burnout and depression among Roman Catholic secular, religious, and monastic clergy, *Pastoral Psychology,* Vol. 47, No. 1, 1998

VITAL: The 2015 physician stress and burnout survey, *VITAL WorkLife and Cejka Search*

Sources for Chapter Two: How Does Burnout Happen?

American Psychological Association. (nd). Stress effects on the body. Retrieved February 27, 2017, from http://www.apa.org/helpcenter/ stress-body.aspx

Brooks, K. A., & Carter, J. G. (2013). Overtraining, exercise, and adrenal insufficiency. *Journal of Novel Physiotherapies, 16*(3). doi:10.4172/2165-7025.1000125

Durning, S. J., Costanzo, M., Artino, A. R., Dyrbye, L. N., Beckman, T. J., & Schuwirth, L. (2013). Functional neuroimaging correlates of burnout among internal medicine residents and faculty members. *Frontiers in Psychiatry, 4.* doi:10.3389/fpsyt.2013.00131

Golkar, A., Johansson, E., Kasahara, M., Osika, W., Perski, A., & Savic, I. (n.d.). The influence of work-related chronic stress on the regulation of emotion and on functional connectivity in the brain. Retrieved May 04, 2017, from http://journals.plos.org/plosone/ article?id=10.1371%2Fjournal.pone.0104550. PLOS One Open Access, 9:9, e104550

Kakiashvili, T., Leszek, J., & Rutkowski, K. (2013). The medical perspective on burnout. *International Journal of Occupational Medicine and Environmental Health, 26*(3), 401–412. doi:10.2478/s13382-013-0093-3

Leiter, M. P., & Maslach, C. (2003). Areas of worklife: A structured approach to organizational predictors of job burnout. In *Emotional and Physiological Processes and Positive Intervention Strategies: Research in Occupational Stress and Well Being* (Vol. 3, pp. 91–134). Kidlington, Oxford, UK: Elsevier Ltd. doi:0.1016/S1479-3555(03)03003-8

Lennartsson, A., Sjörs, A., Währborg, P., Ljung, T., & Jonsdottir, I. H.

(2015). Burnout and hypocortisolism: A matter of severity? A study on ACTH and cortisol responses to acute psychosocial stress. *Frontiers in Psychiatry, 6.* doi:10.3389/fpsyt.2015.00008

Marchand, A., Durand, P., Juster, R., & Lupien, S. J. (2014). Workers' psychological distress, depression, and burnout symptoms: associations with diurnal cortisol profiles. *Scandinavian Journal of Work, Environment & Health, 40*(3), 305–314. doi:10.5271/sjweh.3417

Maslach, C., & Leiter, M. (2005). Reversing burnout: How to rekindle your passion for your work. *Stanford Social Innovation Review, 3*(4), Winter, 42–49.

Shoji, K., Lesnierowska, M., Smoktunowicz, E., Bock, J., Luszczynska, A., Benight, C. C., & Cieslak, R. (2015). What comes first, job burnout or secondary traumatic stress? Findings from two longitudinal studies from the U.S. and Poland. *Plos One, 10*(8). doi:10.1371/journal.pone.0136730

Vente, W. D., Amsterdam, J. G., Olff, M., Kamphuis, J. H., & Emmelkamp, P. M. (2015). Burnout is associated with reduced parasympathetic activity and reduced HPA axis responsiveness, predominantly in males. *BioMed Research International, 2015,* 1–13. doi:10.1155/2015/431725

Whirledge, S., & Cidlowski, J. A. (2010). Glucocorticoids, stress, and fertility. *Minerva Endocrinology, 35*(2), 109–125.

Sources for Chapter Three: Recognizing Burnout When You See It and Feel It

Britton, A., & Shipley, M. J. (2010). Bored to death? *International Journal of Epidemiology, 39*(2), 370–371. doi:10.1093/ije/dyp404

Dyrbye, L. N., Szydlo, D. W., Downing, S. M., Sloan, J. A., & Shanafelt, T. D. (2010). Development and preliminary psychometric properties of a well-being index for medical students. *BMC Medical Education, 10*(1). doi:10.1186/1472-6920-10-8

Headington Institute. (n.d.). Are you showing signs of burnout? Retrieved May 5, 2017, from http://www.headington-institute.org/files/are-you-showing-signs-of-burnout-for-emerg-responders_48145.pdf

Maslach, C., & Jackson, S. E. (1984). Burnout in organizational settings. In S. Oskamp (Ed.), Applied Social Psychology Annual (Vol. 5, pp. 133–153). Beverly Hills, CA: Sage.

Melchers, M. C., Plieger, T., Meermann, R., & Reuter, M. (2015).

Differentiating burnout from depression: Personality matters! *Frontiers in Psychiatry, 6.* doi:10.3389/fpsyt.2015.00113

Montero-Marín, J., Skapinakis, P., Araya, R., Gili, M., & García-Campayo, J. (2011). Towards a brief definition of burnout syndrome by subtypes: Development of the "Burnout Clinical Subtypes Questionnaire" (BCSQ-12). *Health and Quality of Life Outcomes, 9*(1), 74. doi:10.1186/1477-7525-9-74

Montero-Marín, J., Araya, R., Blazquez, B. O., Skapinakis, P., Vizcaino, V. M., & García-Campayo, J. (2012). Understanding burnout according to individual differences: ongoing explanatory power evaluation of two models for measuring burnout types. *BMC Public Health, 12*(1). doi:10.1186/1471-2458-12-922

Montero-Marín, J., Prado-Abril, J., Carrasco, J. M., Asensio-Martínez, Á, Gascón, S., & García-Campayo, J. (2013). Causes of discomfort in the academic workplace and their associations with the different burnout types: a mixed-methodology study. *BMC Public Health, 13,* 1240th ser. doi: 10.1186/1471-2458-13-1240

Smith, M., Segal, J., Robertson, L., & Segal, R. (2016, December). Burnout prevention and recovery. Retrieved January 30, 2017, from https://www.helpguide.org/articles/stress/preventing-burnout.htm The table "Stress vs. Burnout," and the list of Behavioral Warning Signs of Burnout used by permission.

Valcour, M. (2016, June 20). Steps to take when you're starting to feel burned out. Retrieved January 30, 2017, from *Harvard Business Review*: https://hbr.org/2016/06/steps-to-take-when-youre-starting-to-feel-burned-out

West, C. P., Dyrbye, L. N., Sloan, J. A., & Shanafelt, T. D. (2009). Single item measures of emotional exhaustion and depersonalization are useful for assessing burnout in medical professionals. *Journal of General Internal Medicine, 24*(12), 1318–1321. doi:10.1007/s11606-009-1129-z

West, C. P., Dyrbye, L. N., Satele, D. V., Sloan, J. A., & Shanafelt, T. D. (2012). Concurrent validity of single-item measures of emotional exhaustion and depersonalization in burnout assessment. *Journal of General Internal Medicine, 27*(11), 1445–1452. doi:10.1007/s11606-012-2015-7

Wurm, W., Vogel, K., Holl, A., Ebner, C., Bayer, D., Mörkl, S. . . . Hofmann, P. (2016). Depression-burnout overlap in physicians. *Plos One, 11*(3). doi:10.1371/journal.pone.0149913

Sources for Chapter Four: What Stands Between You and Burnout: Five Key Areas

Loomis, M. A., (2015). Not just a personal problem, practitioner burnout is a public health issue. Retrieved December 20, 2015 from www. holisticprimarycare.net/topics/topics-o-z/psyche-somea-spirit/ 1687-not-just-a-personal-problem-practitioner-burnout-is-apublic-health-issue.html. Online Journal: *Holistic Primary Care*

Sources for Chapter Five: Where Are You Strong? Where Are You Vulnerable? Your Burnout Shield Self-Tests

Chapter Five: Multi-Area Sources
Note: The information in the studies and reviews listed in this section apply to more than one of the Burnout Shield's five key areas.

Adshead, G. (2005). Healing ourselves: ethical issues in the care of sick doctors. *Advances in Psychiatric Treatment, 11*(5), 330–337. doi:10.1192/apt.11.5.330

Awa, W. L., Plaumann, M., & Walter, U. (2010). Burnout prevention: A review of intervention programs. *Patient Education and Counseling, 78*(2), 184–190. doi:10.1016/j.pec.2009.04.008

Balch, C. M., Freischlag, J. A., & Shanafelt, T. D. (2009). Stress and burnout among surgeons. *Archives of Surgery, 144*(4), 371–376. doi:10.1001/archsurg.2008.575

Bruyneel, L., Heede, K. V., Diya, L., Aiken, L., & Sermeus, W. (2009). Predictive validity of the International Hospital Outcomes Study Questionnaire: An RN4CAST pilot study. *Journal of Nursing Scholarship, 41*(2), 202–210. doi:10.1111/j.1547-5069.2009.01272.x

Center for Mental Health in Schools at UCLA. (2015). Understanding and minimizing staff burnout. An introductory packet. (rev 2015). Retrieved May 05, 2017, from http://smhp.psych.ucla.edu/pdfdocs/ burnout/burn1.pdf

Cohen-Katz, J., Wiley, S. D., Capuano, T., Baker, D. M., & Shapiro, S. (2005). The effects of mindfulness-based stress reduction on nurse stress and burnout, Part II. *Holistic Nursing Practice, 19*(1), 26–35.

Cohen-Katz, J., Wiley, S., Capuano, T., Baker, D. M., Deitrick, L., & Shapiro, S. (2005). The Effects of mindfulness-based stress reduction on nurse stress and burnout, part III. *Holistic Nursing Practice, 19*(2), 78–86. doi:10.1097/00004650-200503000-00009

Dewe, P. J., O'Driscoll, M. P., & Cooper, G. L. (2012). Theories of Psychological Stress at Work. In *Handbook of Occupational Health and Wellness* (VII ed., pp. 23–38). Heidelberg, Germany: Springer.

Dyrbye, L. N., Thomas, M. R., & Shanafelt, T. D. (2005). Medical student distress: Causes, consequences, and proposed solutions. *Mayo Clinic Proceedings, 80*(12), 1613–1622. doi:10.4065/80.12.1613

Dyrbye, L. N., Power, D. V., Massie, F. S., Eacker, A., Harper, W., Thomas, M. R. . . . Shanafelt, T. D. (2010). Factors associated with resilience to and recovery from burnout: a prospective, multi-institutional study of US medical students. *Medical Education, 44*(10), 1016–1026. doi:10.1111/j.1365-2923.2010.03754.x

Faw, L. (2011, November 11). Why millennial women are burning out at work by 30. *Forbes.* Retrieved May 5, 2017, from https://www.forbes.com/sites/larissafaw/2011/11/11/why-millennial-women-are-burning-out-at-work-by-30/#27800251664d

Friedman, I. A. (2000). Burnout in teachers: Shattered dreams of impeccable professional performance. *Journal of Clinical Psychology, 56*(5), 595–606. doi:10.1002/(sici)1097-4679(200005)56:5<595::aid-jclp2>3.0.co;2-q

Hätinen, M., Mäkikangas, A., Kinnunen, U., & Pekkonen, M. (2013). Recovery from burnout during a one-year rehabilitation intervention with six-month follow-up: Associations with coping strategies. *International Journal of Stress Management, 20*(4), 364–390. doi:10.1037/a0034286

Jackson-Jordan, E. A. (2013). Clergy burnout and resilience: A review of the literature. *Journal of Pastoral Care Counseling, 67*(1), 1–5. doi:10.1177/154230501306700103

Lee, R. T., Seo, B., Hladkyj, S., Lovell, B. L., & Schwartzmann, L. (2013). Correlates of physician burnout across regions and specialties: a meta-analysis. *Human Resources for Health, 11*(1). doi:10.1186/1478-4491-11-48

Maslach, C., & Leiter, M. P. (2016). Understanding the burnout experience: recent research and its implications for psychiatry. *World Psychiatry, 15*(2), 103–111. doi:10.1002/wps.20311

Michie, S. (2003). Reducing work related psychological ill health and sickness absence: a systematic literature review. *Occupational and Environmental Medicine, 60*(1), 3–9. doi:10.1136/oem.60.1.3

Pisanti, R., Doef, M. V., Maes, S., Meier, L. L., Lazzari, D., & Violani, C. (2016). How changes in psychosocial job characteristics impact burnout in nurses: A longitudinal analysis. *Frontiers in Psychology, 7,* 1085. doi:10.3389/fpsyg.2016.01082

Roberts, G. A. (1997). Prevention of burn-out. *Advances in Psychiatric Treatment, 3,* 282–289. doi:10.1192/apt..5.282

Schwarz, T., & Porath, C. (2014, May 30). Why you hate work. *The New York Times Sunday Review.* Retrieved from https://www.nytimes.com/2014/06/01/opinion/sunday/why-you-hate-work.html

Shanafelt, T. D., Dyrbye, L. N., & West, C. P. (2017). Addressing physician burnout: the way forward. *JAMA, 317*(9), 901. doi:10.1001/jama.2017.0076

Shepard, B. C. (2013). Between harm reduction, loss and wellness: on the occupational hazards of work. *Harm Reduction Journal, 10*(5), 5. doi:10.1186/1477-7517-10-5

Shimizutani, M., Odagiri, Y., Ohya, Y., Shimomitsu, T., Kristensen, T. S., Maruta, T., & Iimori, M. (2008). Relationship of nurse burnout with personality characteristics and coping behaviors. *Industrial Health, 46*(4), 326–335. doi:10.2486/indhealth.46.326

Stringfellow Otey, B. (2014). Buffering burnout: Preparing the online generation for the occupational hazards of the legal profession. Retrieved May 5, 2017, from http://www.law.usc.edu/why/students/orgs/ilj/assets/docs/24-1-StringfellowOtey.pdf

UC Davis. (n.d.). Overcoming the challenges of medical school: resources for families. Retrieved May 5, 2017, from https://www.ucdmc.ucdavis.edu/mdprogram/student_wellness/pdfs/Student-Wellness-Trifold.pdf

Chapter Five: More Sources for the Self-Care Self-Test

Bretland, R. J., & Thorsteinsson, E. B. (2015). Reducing workplace burnout: the relative benefits of cardiovascular and resistance exercise. *PeerJ, 3.* doi:10.7717/peerj.891

Daly, B., & Morton, L. L. (2011). The end of leisure: Are preferred leisure activities contraindicated for education-related stress/anxiety reduction? *Education Research International, 2011,* 1–10. doi:10.1155/2011/471838

Díaz-Rodríguez, L., Arroyo-Morales, M., Cantarero-Villanueva, I., Férnandez-Lao, C., Polley, M., & Fernández-De-Las-Peñas, C. (2011).

The application of Reiki in nurses diagnosed with burnout syndrome has beneficial effects on concentration of salivary IgA and blood pressure. *Revista Latino-Americana de Enfermagem, 19*(5), 1132–1138. doi:10.1590/s0104-11692011000500010

Isaksson Ro, K. E., Tyssen, R., Gude, T., & Aasland, O. G. (2012). Will sick leave after a counselling intervention prevent later burnout? A 3-year follow-up study of Norwegian doctors. *Scandinavian Journal of Public Health, 40*(3), 278–285. doi:10.1177/1403494812443607

Isaksson Ro, K. E., Gude, T., Tyssen, R., & Aasland, O. G. (2008). Counselling for burnout in Norwegian doctors: one year cohort study. *BMJ Online First, 337*(Nov11 3). doi:10.1136/bmj.a2004

It's not too early for medical students to think about burnout. (2012, October 1). Retrieved May 4, 2017, from https://www.usnews.com/education/blogs/medical-school-admissions-doctor/2012/10/01/its-not-too-early-for-medical-students-to-think-about-physician-burnout

Korczak, D., Wastian, M., & Schneider, M. (2012, June 14). Therapy of the burnout syndrome. Retrieved May 5, 2017, from https://www.ncbi.nlm.nih.gov/pmc/articles/PMC3434360/. *GMS Health Technol Assess.* 8: Doc05. doi: 10.3205/hta000103

Litscher, G., Liu, C., Wang, L., Wang, L., Li, Q., Shi, G. . . . Wang, X. (2013). Improvement of the dynamic responses of heart rate variability patterns after needle and laser acupuncture treatment in patients with burnout syndrome: A transcontinental comparative study. *Evidence-Based Complementary and Alternative Medicine, 2013,* 1–6. doi:10.1155/2013/128721

McManus, I. C., Jonvik, H., Richards, P., & Paice, E. (2011). Vocation and avocation: leisure activities correlate with professional engagement, but not burnout, in a cross-sectional survey of UK doctors. *BMC Medicine, 9*(100). doi:10.1186/1741-7015-9-100

Moyle, W., Cooke, M., O'Dwyer, S. T., Murfield, J., Johnston, A., & Sung, B. (2013). The effect of foot massage on long-term care staff working with older people with dementia: a pilot, parallel group, randomized controlled trial. *BMC Nursing, 12*(5). doi:10.1186/1472-6955-12-5

Rodriguez, J. E., Welch, T. J., Saunders, C., & Edwards, J. C. (2014). Students' perceptions of the impact a creative arts journal has on their medical education. *Family Medicine, 45*(8), 569–571.

Shea, J. A., Bellini, L. M., Dinges, D. F., Curtis, M. L., Tao, Y., Zhu, J. . . . Volpp, K. G. (2014). Impact of protected sleep period for internal medicine interns on overnight call on depression, burnout, and empathy. *Journal of Graduate Medical Education, 6*(2), 256–263. doi:10.4300/jgme-d-13-00241.1

Sonnenschein, M., Sorbi, M. J., Verbraak, M. J., Schaufeli, W. B., Maas, C. J., & Doornen, L. J. (2008). Influence of sleep on symptom improvement and return to work in clinical burnout. *Scandinavian Journal of Work, Environment & Health, 34*(1), 23–32. doi:10.5271/sjweh.1195

Tsai, H. H., Yeh, C. Y., Su, C. T., Chen, C. J., Peng, S. M., & Chen, R. Y. (2013). The effects of exercise program on burnout and metabolic syndrome components in banking and insurance workers. *Industrial Health, 51*(3), 336–346. doi:10.2486/indhealth.2012-0188

Zawadzki, M. J., Smyth, J. M., & Costigan, H. J. (2015). Real-time associations between engaging in leisure and daily health and well-being. *Annals of Behavioral Medicine, 49*(4), 605–615. doi:10.1007/s12160-015-9694-3

Chapter Five: More Sources for the Reflection & Recognition Self-Test

Ambrose, S. C., Rutherford, B. N., Shepherd, C. D., & Tashchian, A. (2014). Boundary spanner multi-faceted role ambiguity and burnout: An exploratory study. *Industrial Marketing Management, 43*(6), 1070–1078. doi:10.1016/j.indmarman.2014.05.020

Costa, E. O., Santos, A., Santos, A. A., Melo, E., & Andrade, T. (2012). Burnout syndrome and associated factors among medical students: a cross-sectional study. *Clinics, 67*(6), 573–579. doi:10.6061/clinics/2012(06)05

Dane, E., & Brummel, B. J. (2014). Examining workplace mindfulness and its relations to job performance and turnover intention. *Human Relations, 67*(1), 105–128. doi:10.1177/0018726713487753

Davis, D. M., & Hayes, J. A. (2011). What are the benefits of mindfulness? A practice review of psychotherapy-related research. *Psychotherapy, 48*(2), 198–208. doi:10.1037/a0022062

Dyrbye, L. N., Massie, F. S., Eacker, A., Harper, W., Power, D., Durning, S. J. . . . Shanafelt, T. D. (2010). Relationship between burnout and professional conduct and attitudes among US medical students. *JAMA, 304*(11), 1173–1180. doi:10.1001/jama.2010.1318

Elder, C., Nidich, S., & Moriarty, F. (2014). Effect of transcendental meditation on employee stress, depression, and burnout: A randomized controlled study. *The Permanente Journal, 18*(1), 19–23. doi:10.7812/tpp/13-102

Employee Job Satisfaction and Engagement: The Road to Economic Recovery (Rep.). (2014, May 7). Retrieved from https://www.shrm.org/hr-today/trends-and-forecasting/research-and-surveys/documents/14-0028%20jobsatengage_report_full_fnl.pdf

Faragher, E. B., Cass, M., & Cooper, C. L. (2005). The relationship between job satisfaction and health: a meta-analysis. *Occupational and Environmental Medicine, 62*(2), 105–112. doi:10.1136/oem.2002.006734

Fisch, M. J. (2012). Buoyancy: A model for self-reflection about stress and burnout in oncology providers. *2012 Educational Book,* E77-E80. Retrieved from http://meetinglibrary.asco.org/sites/meetinglibrary.asco.org/files/Educational%20Book/PDF%20Files/2012/zds00112000e77.pdf. doi: 10.14694/EdBook_AM.2012.32.e77

Frellick, M. (2016, March 9). In physician burnout, connection is protection. Retrieved May 05, 2017, from http://www.medscape.com/viewarticle/860087. *Medscape Medical News > Conference News*

Goetz, K., Loew, T., Hornung, R., Cojocaru, L., Lahmann, C., & Tritt, K. (2013). Primary prevention programme for burnout-endangered teachers: Follow-up effectiveness of a combined group and individual intervention of AFA breathing therapy. *Evidence-Based Complementary and Alternative Medicine, 2013,* 1–8. doi:10.1155/2013/798260

Hernandez, W., Luthanen, A., Ramsel, D., & Osatuke, K. (2015). The mediating relationship of self-awareness on supervisor burnout and workgroup civility & psychological safety: A multilevel path analysis. *Burnout Research, 2*(1), 36–49. doi:10.1016/j.burn.2015.02.002

Khamisa, N., Peltzer, K., & Oldenburg, B. (2013). Burnout in relation to specific contributing factors and health outcomes among nurses: A systematic review. *International Journal of Environmental Research and Public Health, 10*(6), 2214–2240. doi:10.3390/ijerph10062214

Kjeldstadli, K., Tyssen, R., Finset, A., Hem, E., Gude, T., Gronvold, N. T. . . . Vaglum, P. (2006). Life satisfaction and resilience in medical school — a six-year longitudinal, nationwide and comparative study. *BMC Medical Education, 6*(1). doi:10.1186/1472-6920-6-48

Knudsen, H. K., Roman, P. M., & Abraham, A. J. (2013). Quality of clinical supervision and counselor emotional exhaustion: The potential mediating roles of organizational and occupational commitment. *Journal of Substance Abuse Treatment, 44*(5), 528–533. doi:10.1016/j. jsat.2012.12.003

Leiter, M. P., Frank, E., & Matheson, T. (2009). Values, demands, and burnout: Perspectives from national survey of Canadian physicians. *CFP-MFC Canadian Family Physician, 55*(12), 1224–1225.e6. doi:10.1037/e604522009-001

Lian, P., Sun, Y., Ji, Z., Li, H., & Peng, J. (2014). Moving away from exhaustion: How core self-evaluations influence academic burnout. *PLoS ONE, 9*(1). doi:10.1371/journal.pone.0087152

Shanafelt, T. D. (2009). Enhancing meaning in work. *JAMA, 302*(12), 1338–1340. doi:10.1001/jama.2009.1385

Shepard, B. C. (2013). Between harm reduction, loss and wellness: on the occupational hazards of work. *Harm Reduction Journal, 10*(1), 5. doi:10.1186/1477-7517-10-5

Vibe, M. D., Solhaug, I., Tyssen, R., Friborg, O., Rosenvinge, J. H., Sørlie, T., & Bjørndal, A. (2013). Mindfulness training for stress management: A randomised controlled study of medical and psychology students. *BMC Medical Education, 13*(1). doi:10.1186/1472-6920-13-107

Vilardaga, R., Luoma, J. B., Hayes, S. C., Pistorello, J., Levin, M. E., Hildebrandt, M. J., . . . Bond, F. (2011). Burnout among the addiction counseling workforce: The differential roles of mindfulness and values-based processes and work-site factors. *Journal of Substance Abuse Treatment, 40*(4), 323–335. doi:10.1016/j.jsat.2010.11.015

Wiseman, L., & McKeown, G. (2010, May). Managing yourself: Bringing out the best in your people. Retrieved May 04, 2017, from *Harvard Business Review*, https://hbr.org/2010/05/managing-yourself-bringing-out-the-best-in-your-people

Chapter Five: More Sources for the Capacity Self-Test

Agius, R. M., Blenkin, H., Deary, I. J., Zealley, H. E., & Wood, R. A. (1996). Survey of perceived stress and work demands of consultant doctors. *Occupational and Environmental Medicine, 53*(4), 217–224. doi:10.1136/oem.53.4.217

Aiken, L. H., Sermeus, W., Heede, K. V., Sloane, D. M., Busse, R., McKee, M. . . . Kutney-Lee, A. (2012). Patient safety, satisfaction, and quality of hospital care: cross sectional surveys of nurses and patients in 12 countries in Europe and the United States. *BMJ, 344.* doi: 10.1136/bmj.e1717

Aiken, L. H., Sloane, D., Griffiths, P., Rafferty, A. M., Bruyneel, L., McHugh, M. . . . Sermeus, W. (2016). Nursing skill mix in European hospitals: cross-sectional study of the association with mortality, patient ratings, and quality of care. *BMJ Quality & Safety.* doi:10.1136/bmjqs-2016-005567

Alemany-Martinez, A., Berini-Aytes, L., & Gay-Escoda, C. (2008). The burnout syndrome and associated personality disturbances. The study in three graduate programs in dentistry at the University of Barcelona. *Med Oral Patol Oral Cir Bucal,13*(7), E444-E450.

Backović, D. V., Živojinović, J. I., Maksimović, J., & Maksimović, M. (2012). Gender differences in academic stress and burnout among medical students in final years of education. *Psychiatria Danubina, 24*(2), 175–181.

Baka, L. (2015). Does job burnout mediate negative effects of job demands on mental and physical health in a group of teachers? Testing the energetic process of Job Demands-Resources model. *International Journal of Occupational Medicine and Environmental Health, 28*(2), 335–346. doi:10.13075/ijomeh.1896.00246

Blom, V., Bergström, G., Hallsten, L., Bodin, L., & Svedberg, P. (2012). Genetic susceptibility to burnout in a Swedish twin cohort. *European Journal of Epidemiology, 27*(3), 225–231. doi:10.1007/s10654-012-9661-2

Blom, V., Bodin, L., Bergström, G., Hallsten, L., & Svedberg, P. (2013). The Importance of genetic and shared environmental factors for the associations between job demands, control, support and burnout. *PLoS ONE, 8*(9). doi:10.1371/journal.pone.0075387

Burke, R. J., Matthiesen, S. B., & Pallesen, S. (2006). Workaholism, organizational life and well-being of Norwegian nursing staff. *Career Development International, 11*(5), 463–477. doi:10.1108/13620430610683070

Collier, R. (2012). The "physician personality" and other factors in physician health. *Canadian Medical Association Journal, 184*(18), 1980–1980. doi:10.1503/cmaj.109-4329

Dubois, C., Bentein, K., Mansour, J., Gilbert, F., & Bédard, J. (2013). Why some employees adopt or resist reorganization of work practices in health care: Associations between perceived loss of resources, burnout, and attitudes to change. *International Journal of Environmental Research and Public Health, 11*(1), 187–201. doi:10.3390/ijerph110100187

Finney, C., Stergiopoulos, E., Hensel, J., Bonato, S., & Dewa, C. S. (2013). Organizational stressors associated with job stress and burnout in correctional officers: a systematic review. *BMC Public Health, 13*(1). doi:10.1186/1471-2458-13-82

Gleichgerrcht, E., & Decety, J. (2013). Empathy in clinical practice: How individual dispositions, gender, and experience moderate empathic concern, burnout, and emotional distress in physicians. *PLoS ONE, 8*(4). doi:10.1371/journal.pone.0061526

Glise, K., Ahlborg, G., & Jonsdottir, I. H. (2012). Course of mental symptoms in patients with stress-related exhaustion: does sex or age make a difference? *BMC Psychiatry, 12*(1). doi:10.1186/1471-244x-12-18

Hakanen, J. J., Bakker, A. B., & Jokisaari, M. (2011). A 35-year follow-up study on burnout among Finnish employees. *Journal of Occupational Health Psychology, 16*(3), 345–360. doi:10.1037/a0022903

Holden, R. J., Patel, N. R., Scanlon, M. C., Shalaby, T. M., Arnold, J. M., & Karsh, B. (2010). Effects of mental demands during dispensing on perceived medication safety and employee well-being: A study of workload in pediatric hospital pharmacies. *Research in Social and Administrative Pharmacy, 6*(4), 293–306. doi:10.1016/j.sapharm.2009.10.001

Legrain, A., Eluru, N., & El-Geneidy, A. M. (2015). Am stressed, must travel: The relationship between mode choice and commuting stress. *Transportation Research Part F: Traffic Psychology and Behaviour, 34*, 141–151. doi:10.1016/j.trf.2015.08.001

Leiter, M. P., Day, A., & Price, L. (2015). Attachment styles at work: Measurement, collegial relationships, and burnout. *Burnout Research, 2*(1), 25–35. doi:10.1016/j.burn.2015.02.003

Lucas, J., & Heady, R. P. (2002). Flextime commuters and their driver stress, feelings of time urgency, and commute satisfaction. *J of Business and Psychology, 16*(4), 565–571. doi:10.1023/A:1015402302281

McMurray, Julia E., Mark Linzer, Thomas R. Konrad, Jeffrey Douglas, Richard Shugerman, and Kathleen Nelson. The work lives of women physicians. Results from the Physician Work Life Study. *Journal of General Internal Medicine* 15.6 (2000): 372–80. Web.

Nahrgang, J. D., Morgeson, F. P., & Hofmann, D. A. (2011). Safety at work: A meta-analytic investigation of the link between job demands, job resources, burnout, engagement, and safety outcomes. *Journal of Applied Psychology, 96*(1), 71–94. doi:10.1037/a0021484

Novaco, R. W. (1992). Commuter stress. *Access, 01,* 29–31. Retrieved from http://www.accessmagazine.org/wp-content/uploads/sites/7/2016/07/access01-06-Commuter-Stress.pdf

Pejušković, B., Lečić-Toševski, D., Priebe, S., & Tošković, O. (2011). Burnout syndrome among physicians — the role of personality dimensions and coping strategies. *Psychiatr Danub., 23*(4), 389–395.

Richards, V. (2015, May 27). Commuting for more than 20 minutes makes you 'stressed and cynical'. *Independent.* Retrieved from http://www.independent.co.uk/travel/news-and-advice/commuting-for-more-than-20-minutes-makes-you-stressed-and-cynical-10278874.html

Shanafelt, T. D., Gorringe, G., Menaker, R., Storz, K. A., Reeves, D., Buskirk, S. J. . . . Swensen, S. J. (2015). Impact of organizational leadership on physician burnout and satisfaction. *Mayo Clinic Proceedings, 90*(4), 432–440. doi:10.1016/j.mayocp.2015.01.012

Smith, H. K., & Cunningham, C. J. (2012). Testing work characteristics as mediating factors in the relationship among nurse leadership, burnout, and engagement. *PsycEXTRA Dataset.* doi:10.1037/e577572014-475

Tei, S., Becker, C., Kawada, R., Fujino, J., Jankowski, K. F., Sugihara, G. . . . Takahashi, H. (2014). Can we predict burnout severity from empathy-related brain activity? *Translational Psychiatry, 4*(6). doi:10.1038/tp.2014.34

Wei, M. (2015, January 12). Commuting: "The stress that doesn't pay." *Psychology Today.* Retrieved from https://www.psychologytoday.com/blog/urban-survival/201501/commuting-the-stress-doesnt-pay

West, C. P., Shanafelt, T. D., & Kolars, J. C. (2011). Quality of life, burnout, educational debt, and medical knowledge among internal medicine residents. *JAMA, 306*(9), 952–960. doi:10.1001/jama.2011.1247

Chapter Five: More Sources for the Community Self-Test

Fernet, C., Torrès, O., Austin, S., & St-Pierre, J. (2016). The psychological costs of owning and managing an SME: Linking job stressors, occupational loneliness, entrepreneurial orientation, and burnout. *Burnout Research, 3*(2), 45–53. doi:10.1016/j.burn.2016.03.002

Goncalo, J., Polman, E., & Maslach, C. (2010, May 19). Can confidence come too soon? Collective efficacy, conflict and group performance over time. Retrieved May 4, 2017, from http://digitalcommons.ilr. cornell.edu/cgi/viewcontent.cgi?article=1306&context=articles

Handzel, S. (2016, March 16). Zero tolerance: Stopping nurse bullying begins with leadership. Retrieved May 07, 2017, from http://nursing. onclive.com/publications/oncology-nurse/2017/march-2017/zero-tolerance-stopping-nurse-bullying-begins-with-leadership

Holm, M., Tyssen, R., Stordal, K. I., & Haver, B. (2010, March 16). Self-development groups reduce medical school stress: a controlled intervention study. Retrieved May 04, 2017, from http://bmcmededuc. biomedcentral.com/articles/10.1186/1472-6920-10-23

Love, P. E., Edwards, D. J., & Irani, Z. (2010). Work stress, support, and mental health in construction. *Journal of Construction Engineering and Management, 136*(6), 650–658. doi:10.1061/(ASCE) CO.1943-7862.0000165

Saba, G. W., Villela, T. J., Chen, E., Hammer, H., & Bodenheimer, T. (2012). The myth of the lone physician: Toward a collaborative alternative. *The Annals of Family Medicine, 10*(2), 169–173. doi:10.1370/ afm.1353

Smets, E. M., Visser, M. R., Oort, F. J., Schaufeli, W. B., Hanneke, J., & De Haes, C. (2004). Perceived inequity: Does it explain burnout among medical specialists? *Journal of Applied Social Psychology, 34*(9), 1900–1918. doi:10.1111/j.1559-1816.2004.tb02592.x

Tsai, Y. (2011). Relationship between organizational culture, leadership behavior and job satisfaction. *BMC Health Services Research, 11*(98). doi:10.1186/1472-6963-11-98

Willard-Grace, R., Hessler, D., Rogers, E., Dube, K., Bodenheimer, T., & Grumbach, K. (2014). Team structure and culture are associated with lower burnout in primary care. *The Journal of the American Board of Family Medicine, 27*(2), 229–238. doi:10.3122/jabfm.2014.02.130215

Yoon, J. D., Rasinski, K. A., & Curlin, F. A. (2010). Conflict and emotional exhaustion in obstetrician-gynaecologists: a national survey. *Journal of Medical Ethics, 36*(12), 731–735. doi:10.1136/jme.2010.037762

Chapter Five: More Sources for the Coping Skills Self-Test

Angermeier, I., Dunford, B. B., Boss, A. D., & Boss, R. W. (2009). The impact of participative management perceptions on customer service, medical errors, burnout, and turnover intentions. *J Healthc Manag. , 54*(2), 1217–40.

Barnard, L. K., & Curry, J. F. (2011). The relationship of clergy burnout to self-compassion and other personality dimensions. *Pastoral Psychology, 61*(2), 149–163. doi:10.1007/s11089-011-0377-0

Beebe, R., & Frisch, N. (2009). Development of the differentiation of self and role inventory for nurses (DSRI-RN): A tool to measure internal dimensions of workplace stress. *Nursing Outlook, 57*(5), 240–245. doi:10.1016/j.outlook.2009.04.001

Biglan, A., Layton, G. L., Jones, L. B., Hankins, M., & Rusby, J. C. (2011). The value of workshops on psychological flexibility for early childhood special education staff. *Topics in Early Childhood Special Education, 32*(4), 196–210. doi:10.1177/0271121411425191

Bigos, S. J., Battié, M. C., Spengler, D. M., Fisher, L. D., Fordyce, W. E., Hansson, T. H. . . . Wortley, M. D. (1991). A prospective study of work perceptions and psychosocial factors affecting the report of back injury. *Spine, 16*(1), 1–6. doi:10.1097/00007632-199101000-00001

Carver, C. S., Scheier, M. F., & Weintraub, J. K. (1989). Assessing coping strategies: A theoretically based approach. *Journal of Personality and Social Psychology, 56*(2), 267–283. doi:10.1037//0022-3514.56.2.267

Chullen, C. L. (2014). How does supervisor burnout affect leader-member exchange? A dyadic perspective. *International Business & Economics Research Journal (IBER), 13*(5), 1113–1126. doi:10.19030/iber.v13i5.8777

Erickson, R., & Grove, W. J. (2007). Why emotions matter: Age, agitation, and burnout among registered nurses. *The Online Journal of Issues in Nursing, 13*(1). doi:10.3912/OJIN.Vol13No01PPT01

Estryn-Behar, M., Kaminski, M., Peigne, E., Bonnet, N., Vaichere, E., Gozlan, C. . . . Giorgi, M. (1990). Stress at work and mental health status among female hospital workers. *Occupational and Environmental Medicine, 47*, 20–28. doi:10.1136/oem.47.1.20

Finkelstein, C., Brownstein, A., Scott, C., & Lan, Y. (2007). Anxiety and stress reduction in medical education: an intervention. *Medical Education, 41*(3), 258–264. doi:10.1111/j.1365-2929.2007.02685.x

Flowers, L. K. (2005). The missing curriculum: Experience with emotional competence education and training for premedical and medical students. *JNMA, 97*(9), 1280–1287.

Folkman, S., & Al, E. (1986). Dynamics of a stressful encounter:

Cognitive appraisal, coping, and encounter outcomes. *Journal of Personality and Social Psychology, 50*(5), 992–1003. doi:10.1037//0022-3514.50.5.992

Gan, Y., Shang, J., & Zhang, Y. (2007). Coping flexibility and locus of control as predictors of burnout among Chinese college students. *Social Behavior and Personality: an international journal, 35*(8), 1087–1098. doi:10.2224/sbp.2007.35.8.1087

Heng, K. W. (2014). Teaching and evaluating multitasking ability in emergency medicine residents — what is the best practice? *International Journal of Emergency Medicine, 7*(1). doi:10.1186/s12245-014-0041-4

Kariv, D., & Heiman, T. (2005). Task-oriented versus emotion-oriented coping strategies: The case of college students. *College Student Journal, v39 n1 p72 Mar 2005, 39*(1), 72–85.

Kerfoot, K. M. (2013). Are you tired? Overcoming leadership styles that create leader fatigue. *Nursing Economics, 31*(3), 146–151.

Lemaire, J. B., & Wallace, J. E. (2010). Not all coping strategies are created equal: a mixed methods study exploring physicians' self reported coping strategies. *BMC Health Services Research, 10*(208). doi:10.1186/1472-6963-10-208

Montero-Marin, J., Prado-Abril, J., Demarzo, M. M., Gascon, S., & García-Campayo, J. (2014). Coping with stress and types of burnout: explanatory power of different coping strategies. *PLoS ONE, 9*(2). doi:10.1371/journal.pone.0089090

Prinz, P., Hertrich, K., Hirschfelder, U., & DeZwaan, M. (2012). Burnout, depression and depersonalisation — psychological factors and coping strategies in dental and medical students. *GMS Z Med Ausbikld, 29*(1). doi:10.3205/zma000780

Savage, S. (2005, April 04). Task-oriented versus emotion-oriented coping strategies: The case of college students. Retrieved May 18, 2017, from http://www.redorbit.com/news/health/141147/taskoriented_versus_emotionoriented_coping_strategies_the_case_of_college_students/

Shimizutani, M., Odagiri, Y., Ohya, Y., Shimomitsu, T., Kristensen, T. S., Maruta, T., & Iimori, M. (2008). Relationship of nurse burnout with personality characteristics and coping behaviors. *Industrial Health, 46*(4), 326–335. doi:10.2486/indhealth.46.326

Wilski, M., Chmielewski, B., & Tomczak, M. (2015). Work locus of control and burnout in Polish physiotherapists: The mediating effect of coping styles. *International Journal of Occupational Medicine and Environmental Health, 28*(5), 875–889. doi:10.13075/ijomeh.1896.00287

Sources for Chapter Six: Self-Care: Are You Providing Your Body with the Basic Things that Keep It Going?

Chapter Six: Sleep

Alhola, P., & Polo-Kantola, P. (2007). Sleep deprivation: Impact on cognitive performance. *Neuropsychiatric Disease and Treatment, 3*(5), 553–567.

American Academy of Sleep Medicine. (2008, June 10). Extra sleep improves athletic performance. Retrieved January 20, 2017, from http://www.sciencedaily.com/releases/2008/06/080609071106.htm

American Psychological Association. (2014, February). More sleep would make most Americans happier. Retrieved January 20, 2017, from http://www.apa.org/action/resources/research-in-action/sleep-deprivation.aspx

Caruso, C. C., Hitchcock, E. M., Dick, R. B., Russo, J. M., & Schmit, J. M. (2004, April). Overtime and extended work shifts: recent findings on illnesses, injuries, and health behaviors. Retrieved May 4, 2017, from https://www.cdc.gov/niosh/docs/2004-143/pdfs/2004-143.pdf

Ekstedt, M., Söderström, M., Åkerstedt, T., Nilsson, J., Søndergaard, H., & Aleksander, P. (2006). Disturbed sleep and fatigue in occupational burnout. *Scandinavian Journal of Work, Environment & Health, 32*(2), 121–131. doi:10.5271/sjweh.987

HelpGuide. (n.d.). Not sleeping well? There may be a medical cause. Retrieved January 20, 2017, from http://www.helpguide.org/harvard/medical-causes-of-sleep-problems.htm

Jones, M. (2011, April 15). How Little Sleep Can You Get Away With? *New York Times Magazine*. (Discusses the sleep research of David Dinges, the head of the Sleep and Chronobiology Laboratory at the Hospital at University of Pennsylvania.)

Klein, S. (2013, February 26). Sleep deprivation can change your genes. Retrieved January 20, 2017, from http://www.huffingtonpost.com/2013/02/26/sleep-deprivation-genes_n_2766341.html

Locke, S. (2014, June 10). 7 weird and terrible effects of sleep deprivation. Retrieved January 20, 2017, from http://www.vox.com/2014/6/10/5796676/the-weird-and-terrible-effects-of-sleep-deprivation

Mah, C. D., Mah, K. E., Kezirian, E. J., & Dement, W. C. (2011). The effects of sleep extension on the athletic performance of collegiate basketball players. *Sleep, 34*(07), 943–950. doi:10.5665/sleep.1132

Moller-Levet, C. S., Archer, S. N., Bucca, G., Laing, E. E., Slak, A., Kabiljo, R., . . . Dijk, D. (2013). Effects of insufficient sleep on circadian rhythmicity and expression amplitude of the human blood transcriptome. *Proceedings of the National Academy of Sciences, 110*(12). doi:10.1073/pnas.1217154110

Rajki, M., R.N., C.N.P. (2012, March 18). Sleep problems in older adults. Retrieved January 20, 2017, from http://occupational-therapy.advanceweb.com/Features/Articles/Sleep-Problems-in-Older-Adults.aspx

Schocker, L. (Ed.). (2015, December 13). Here's a horrifying picture of what sleep loss will do to you. Retrieved January 20, 2017, from http://www.huffingtonpost.com/2014/01/08/sleep-deprivation_n_4557142.html. (Great infographic!)

Smit, B. W. (2015). Successfully leaving work at work: The self-regulatory underpinnings of psychological detachment. *Journal of Occupational and Organizational Psychology, 89*(3), 493–514. doi:10.1111/joop.12137

Stanford University Press Release. (1996, January). Stanford researchers suggest how sleep re-charges the brain. Retrieved January 20, 2017, from http://news.stanford.edu/pr/96/960116sleep.html

Söderström, M., Jeding, K., Ekstedt, M., Perski, A., & Åkerstedt, T. (2012). Insufficient sleep predicts clinical burnout. *Journal of Occupational Health Psychology, 17*(2), 175–183. doi:10.1037/a0027518

Thomée, S., Eklöf, M., Gustafsson, E., Nilsson, R., & Hagberg, M. (2007). Prevalence of perceived stress, symptoms of depression and sleep disturbances in relation to information and communication technology (ICT) use among young adults – an explorative prospective study. *Computers in Human Behavior, 23*(3), 1300–1321. doi:10.1016/j.chb.2004.12.007

Tierney, J. (2011, August 17). Do you suffer from decision fatigue? Retrieved January 20, 2017, from http://www.nytimes.com/2011/08/21/magazine/do-you-suffer-from-decision-fatigue.html

Chapter Six: Move the Body

Abderrahman, A., Zouhal, H., Chamari, K., Thevenet, D., De Mullenheim, P., Gastinger, S., & Prioux, J. (2013). Effects of recovery mode (active vs. passive) on performance during a short high-intensity interval training program: a longitudinal study. *European Journal of Applied Physiology and Occupational Physiology, 113*(6), 1373–1383. doi: 10.1007/s00421-012-2556-9

Crowley, C., & Lodge, H. S., M.D. (2004). *Younger next year: a guide to living like 50 until you're 80 and beyond.* New York: Workman Pub.

Chapter Six: See a Doctor

Albrecht, S. (2014, February 7). Why don't employees use EAP services? Retrieved January 20, 2017, from https://www.psychologytoday.com/blog/the-act-violence/201402/why-dont-employees-use-eap-services

National Suicide Prevention Lifeline. (n.d.). National Suicide Prevention Lifeline [Digital image]. Retrieved from http://www.suicidepreventionlifeline.org/. Used by permission.

Renter, E. (2015, June 25). 5 Tips for navigating medical care without health insurance. Retrieved January 20, 2017, from http://health.usnews.com/health-news/health-insurance/articles/2015/06/25/5-tips-for-navigating-medical-care-without-health-insurance

Tolar, T. (2009, April 27). 5 Places to check out medical care for the uninsured. Retrieved January 20, 2017, from http://www.wisebread.com/5-places-to-check-out-medical-care-for-the-uninsured

Chapter Six: Depression

Barnard, C., M.D. (2015, February 27). Foods that fight depression. Retrieved January 20, 2017, from http://www.pcrm.org/nbBlog/index.php/foods-that-fight-depression

Goldberg, J. (Ed.). (2016, August 13). Sleep deprivation and depression: What's the Link? Retrieved January 20, 2017, from http://www.webmd.com/depression/guide/depression-sleep-disorder#1

Greger, M., M.D. (2015, September 18). Plant-based diets for improved mood and productivity. Retrieved January 20, 2017, from http://nutritionfacts.org/video/plant-based-diets-for-improved-mood-and-productivity/

Heesch, K. C., Gellecum, Y. R., Burton, N. W., Uffelen, J. G., & Brown, W. J. (2015). Physical activity, walking, and quality of life in women with depressive symptoms. *American Journal of Preventive Medicine, 48*(3), 281–291. doi:10.1016/j.amepre.2014.09.030

Iliades, C., MD. (2011, July 11). Asking for help when you're depressed.

Retrieved January 20, 2017, from http://www.everydayhealth.com/hs/major-depression/ask-for-help/

Mayo Clinic Staff. (2014, April 15). Post-traumatic stress disorder (PTSD). Retrieved January 20, 2017, from http://www.mayoclinic.org/diseases-conditions/post-traumatic-stress-disorder/basics/definition/con-20022540

Neumann, J. (2015, January 30). Regular walking can help ease depression. Retrieved January 20, 2017, from http://www.scientificamerican.com/article/regular-walking-can-help-ease-depression/

Publications, H. H. (2009, June). Exercise and depression. Retrieved January 20, 2017, from http://www.health.harvard.edu/mind-and-mood/exercise-and-depression-report-excerpt

Chapter Six: Work/Life Separation & Vacations

Della Costa, C. (2016, July 04). Top 5 reasons Americans don't use their vacation days. Retrieved January 20, 2017, from http://www.cheatsheet.com/money-career/the-top-5-reasons-people-dont-use-their-vacation-days.html/?a=viewall

Etzion, D. (2003). Annual vacation: Duration of relief from job stressors and burnout. *Anxiety, Stress & Coping, 16*(2), 213–226. doi:10.1080/1061580021000069425

GfK Public Affairs & Corporate Communications, & US Travel Association. (2014, August). Overwhelmed America: Why don't we use our earned leave? Retrieved January 20, 2017, from http://www.projecttimeoff.com/research/overwhelmed-america

GfK Public Affairs & Corporate Communications, & US Travel Association. (2016). The state of American vacation 2016: How vacation became a casualty of our work culture. Retrieved January 20, 2017, from http://www.projecttimeoff.com/sites/default/files/PTO_SoAV%20Report_FINAL.pdf (Source of table: "Reasons Time is Left on the Table.")

Scribner, H. (2014, August 20). 7 benefits of taking vacation time. Retrieved January 20, 2017, from http://national.deseretnews.com/article/2169/7-benefits-of-taking-vacation-time.html

Soukup, R. (2016, March 07). 25 Awesome staycation ideas. Retrieved January 20, 2017, from http://www.livingwellspendingless.com/2014/03/07/staycation-ideas/

Tugend, A. (2008, June 8). Take a vacation, for your health's sake. *New*

York Times. Retrieved January 20, 2017, from http://www.nytimes.com/2008/06/08/business/worldbusiness/08iht-07shortcuts.13547623.html

Westman, M., & Eden, D. (1997). Effects of a respite from work on burnout: Vacation relief and fade-out. *Journal of Applied Psychology, 82*(4), 516–527. doi:10.1037//0021-9010.82.4.516

Westman, M., & Etzion, D. (2001). The impact of vacation and job stress on burnout and absenteeism. *Psychology & Health, 16*(5), 595–606. doi:10.1080/08870440108405529

Chapter Six: Addiction

Sinha, R. (2008). Chronic Stress, Drug Use, and Vulnerability to Addiction. Annals of the New York Academy of Sciences, 1141(1), 105–130. doi:10.1196/annals.1441.030

Sources for Chapter Seven: Reflection & Recognition: Engage Your Brain's Most Powerful Reward Circuits

Achor, S. (2010). *The happiness advantage: the seven principles of positive psychology that fuel success and performance at work.* New York: Broadway Books.

Beshai, S., McAlpine, L., Weare, K., & Kuyken, W. (2015). A Non-randomised feasibility trial assessing the efficacy of a mindfulness-based intervention for teachers to reduce stress and improve well-being. *Mindfulness, 7*(1), 198–208.

Blouin-Hudon, E. C., & Pychyl, T. A. (2015). Experiencing the temporally extended self: Initial support for the role of affective states, vivid mental imagery, and future self-continuity in the prediction of academic procrastination. *Personality and Individual Differences, 86,* 50–56. doi:10.1016/j.paid.2015.06.003

Flook, L., Goldberg, S. B., Pinger, L., Bonus, K., & Davidson, R. J. (2013). Mindfulness for teachers: A pilot study to assess effects on stress, burnout, and teaching efficacy. *Mind, Brain, and Education, 7*(3), 182–195.

Frederickson, B., PhD, & PEP Lab - Positive Emotions and Psychophysiology Laboratory website, University of North Carolina at Chapel Hill. (2014). PEP Lab. Retrieved January 20, 2017, from http://www.unc.edu/peplab/research.html. See section, "The broaden and build theory of positive emotions."

Genly, B. (2016, July 27). Gratitude and finding meaning. Retrieved

January 20, 2017, from http://www.burnout-solutions.com/gratitude-and-finding-meaning/. Portions of this chapter previously appeared in this blog post. Used by permission.

Hülsheger, U. R., Alberts, H. J., Feinholdt, A., & Lang, J. W. (2013). Benefits of mindfulness at work: The role of mindfulness in emotion regulation, emotional exhaustion, and job satisfaction. *Journal of Applied Psychology, 98*(2), 310–325.

Krasner, M. S., Epstein, R. M., Beckman, H., Suchman, A. L., Chapman, B., Mooney, C. J., & Quill, T. E. (2009). Association of an educational program in mindful communication with burnout, empathy, and attitudes among primary care physicians. *JAMA, 302*(12), 1284–1293. doi:10.1001/jama.2009.1384

Luken, M., & Sammons, A. (2016). Systematic review of mindfulness practice for reducing job burnout. *American Journal of Occupational Therapy, 70*(2). doi:10.5014/ajot.2016.016956

Lyubomirsky, S. (2008). *The how of happiness: a scientific approach to getting the life you want.* New York: Penguin Press.

Matthias, J., Narayanan, J., & Chaturvedi, S. (2014). Leading mindfully: two studies of the influence of supervisor trait mindfulness on employee well- being and performance. *Mindfulness, 5*(1), 36–45. Retrieved from http://ink.library.smu.edu.sg/lkcsb_research/3320

Montero-Marin, J., Monticelli, F., Casas, M., Roman, A., Tomas, I., Gili, M., & Garcia-Campayo, J. (2011). Burnout syndrome among dental students: a short version of the "Burnout Clinical Subtype Questionnaire" adapted for students (BCSQ-12-SS). *BMC Medical Education, 11*(103). doi:10.1186/1472-6920-11-103

Montero-Marin, J., Tops, M., Manzanera, R., Demarzo, M. M., Mon, M. Á, & García-Campayo, J. (2015). Mindfulness, resilience, and burnout subtypes in primary care physicians: The possible mediating role of positive and negative affect. *Frontiers in Psychology, 6*, 1895th ser. doi:10.3389/fpsyg.2015.01895

Scherer, L. L., Allen, J. A., & Harp, E. R. (2016). Grin and bear it: An examination of volunteers' fit with their organization, burnout and spirituality. *Burnout Research, 3*(1), 1–10. doi:10.1016/j.burn.2015.10.003

Swift, J. K., & J. L. (2015, July 01). A Multi-site study of mindfulness training for therapists. *Society for the Advancement of Psychotherapy.* Retrieved January 30, 2017, from http://societyforpsychotherapy.org/a-multi-site-study-of-mindfulness-training-for-therapists/

Sources for Chapter Eight: Capacity: Check the Lay of the Land

Blouin-Hudon, E. C., & Pychyl, T. A. (2016). A mental imagery intervention to increase future self-continuity and reduce procrastination. *Applied Psychology*. doi:10.1111/apps.12088

Dewey, C. M., & Swiggart, W. H. (2017, May 4). *The health and wellness of physicians: Managing stress, burnout and energy*. Lecture presented at Department of Pediatric Grand Rounds in Vanderbilt University School of Medicine. PowerPoint slides retrieved May 5, 2017, from http://www.mc.vanderbilt.edu/documents/cph/files/Professional Health&Wellness_ManagingStressand%20Burnout_2012.pdf

Genly, B. (2016, July 29). Why say no anyway? Retrieved January 20, 2017, from http://www.burnout-solutions.com/why-say-no-anyway/ (Parts of this chapter first appeared, in a somewhat different form, in this blog post. Used by permission.)

Genly, B. (2016, March 17). How guilt & wishful thinking kill fun & increase burnout. Retrieved January 20, 2017, from http://www.burnout-solutions.com/how-guilt-and-wishful-thinking-kill-fun-and-increase-burnout/ (Parts of this chapter first appeared, in a somewhat different form, in this blog post. Used by permission.)

McGonigal, J. (2010, February). Gaming can make a better world. Retrieved February 02, 2017, from https://www.ted.com/talks/jane_mcgonigal_gaming_can_make_a_better_world

Oettingen, G. (2015). *Rethinking Positive thinking: the new science of motivation*. Penguin Group US.

Scott. (2014, November 17). Warren Buffett's 5-step process for prioritizing true success. Retrieved January 20, 2017, from http://liveyourlegend.net/warren-buffetts-5-step-process-for-prioritizing-true-success-and-why-most-people-never-do-it/.

(This attribution has been widely quoted elsewhere. However, this strategy has been attributed to other business leaders as well, such as Lee Iacocca. Beth has also encountered a version of this strategy in: Attwood, Janet Brae, and Attwood, Chris. The passion test: The effortless path to discovering your destiny. 2007, Penguin.)

Sharpe, L. (2013, August 06). So you think you know why animals play . . . Retrieved January 20, 2017, from https://blogs.scientificamerican.com/guest-blog/so-you-think-you-know-why-animals-play/

Suttie, J. (2015, January 12). Four ways music strengthens social bonds.

Retrieved January 20, 2017, from http://greatergood.berkeley.edu/article/item/four_ways_music_strengthens_social_bonds

U.S. Equal Opportunity Employment Commission. (n.d.). Facts about retaliation. Retrieved February 15, 2017, from https://www.eeoc.gov/laws/types/facts-retal.cfm

Urist, J. (2014, September 24). What the marshmallow test really teaches about self-control. Retrieved January 20, 2017, from http://www.theatlantic.com/health/archive/2014/09/what-the-marshmallow-test-really-teaches-about-self-control/380673/

Sources for Chapter Nine: Community: Reconnect, Ask for Help, Get Perspective

Chapter Nine: Prevention/Promotion—Motivational Styles

Brockner, J., & Higgins, E. T. (2001). Regulatory Focus Theory: Implications for the Study of Emotions at Work. Organizational Behavior and Human Decision Processes, 86(1), 35–66. doi:10.1006/obhd.2001.2972

Grant, H., & Higgins, E. T. (2014, July 31). Do you play to win-or to not lose? Retrieved February 06, 2017, from https://hbr.org/2013/03/do-you-play-to-win-or-to-not-lose Also published in Harvard Business Review, March 2013 issue.

Halvorson, H. G., & Higgins, E. T. (2013). *Focus: use different ways of seeing the world for success and influence.* New York: Hudson Street Press.

Chapter Nine: Finding a Mentor, Dealing with Stigma

Bender Phelps, S. (2015, May 06). 10 Tips on how to be a great mentoring partner. Retrieved January 20, 2017, from http://susanbenderphelps.com/news/10-tips-on-how-to-be-a-great-mentoring-partner/

Dziura, J. (2015, October 03). How to ask for help in your career. Retrieved January 20, 2017, from http://www.slideshare.net/JenDziura/how-to-ask-for-help-in-you-career [Slideshow]

Makovsky, K. (n.d.). Communications in high stress environments. *Forbes.* Retrieved from http://www.forbes.com/sites/kenmakovsky/2013/10/03/1159/

Mowry, D., & Rolstad, T. (2015). *No, really, we want you to laugh: Mental illness and stand-up comedy: Transforming lives.* Portland, OR: Alagon Press.

Qian, J., Han, Z., Wang, H., Li, X., & Wang, Q. (2014). Power distance and mentor-protégé relationship quality as moderators of the relationship between informal mentoring and burnout: evidence from China. *International Journal of Mental Health Systems, 8*(51). doi:10.1186/1752-4458-8-51

Vogel, D. L., & Wade, N. G. (2009, January). Stigma and help-seeking. Retrieved January 20, 2017, from https://thepsychologist.bps.org.uk/volume-22/edition-1/stigma-and-help-seeking

Chapter Nine: Positivity

Fredrickson, B. L. (2013). Updated thinking on positivity ratios. *American Psychologist, 68*(9), 814–822. doi:10.1037/a0033584

Otaṣuke, K., Leiter, M., Belton, L., Dyrenforth, S., & Ramsel, D. (2013). Civility, respect and engagement at the workplace (CREW): a national organization development program at the Department of Veterans Affairs. *Journal of Management Policies and Practices, 1*(2), 25–34. doi:DOI: 10.15640/jmpp

Work Engagement. (2017). Four Principles for groups to build on the positive. Retrieved February 17, 2017, from http://workengagement.com/index.php/crew/crew-faq/5-op/civ/124-four-principles-for-groups-to-build-on-the-positive

Sources for Chapter Ten: Coping Skills: Rethink Your Reactions

Bakker, A. B., Demerouti, E., & Schaufeli, W. B. (2005). The crossover of burnout and work engagement among working couples. *Human Relations, 58*(5), 661–689. doi:10.1177/0018726705055967

Bakker, A. B., & Heuven, E. (2006). Emotional dissonance, burnout, and in-role performance among nurses and police officers. *International Journal of Stress Management, 13*(4), 423–440. doi:10.1037/1072-5245.13.4.423

Barber, L. K., Taylor, S. G., Burton, J. P., & Bailey, S. F. (2017). A self-regulatory perspective of work-to-home undermining spillover/crossover: Examining the roles of sleep and exercise. *Journal of Applied Psychology.* doi:10.1037/apl0000019 Feb 2 [Epub ahead of print]

Katie, B. (2015, September 06). Do the work. Retrieved February 06, 2017, from http://thework.com/en/do-work

MacMillan, A. (2017, February 9). You need to deal with your work stress. Here's how. Retrieved February 10, 2017, from http://time.com/4665623/exercise-work-stress-sleep/

McNamara on February 2, 2012, C. (2012, February 02). Basic guidelines to reframing—to seeing things differently. Retrieved February 06, 2017, from http://managementhelp.org/blogs/personal-and-professional-coaching/2012/02/02/basic-guidelines-to-reframing-to-seeing-things-differently/

Nabi, H., Singh-Manoux, A., Ferrie, J. E., Marmot, M. G., Melchior, M., & Kivimäki, M. (2009). Hostility and depressive mood: results from the Whitehall II prospective cohort study. *Psychological Medicine, 40*(03), 405–413. doi:10.1017/s0033291709990432

Project: Time Off. (2016, November 02). The state of American vacation: How vacation became a casualty of our work culture. Retrieved January 20, 2017, from http://www.projecttimeoff.com/research/state-american-vacation-2016 (Source of table: "Reason Time is Left on the Table," used by permission.)

Rolstad, T. (2016). Celebrate your best bad [Web log post]. First publication: reprinted by permission of the author.

Wikipedia. (2017, February 22). Cynicism (contemporary). Retrieved February 23, 2017, from https://en.wikipedia.org/wiki/Cynicism_(contemporary) Source of the definition of cynicism discussed in this chapter.

Sources for Chapter Eleven: Staying Out of Burnout

Achor, S., & Gielan, M. (2016, October 23). Resilience is about how you recharge, not how you endure. Retrieved January 28, 2017, from https://hbr.org/2016/06/resilience-is-about-how-you-recharge-not-how-you-endure

About the Authors

Marnie Loomis, ND, is a naturopathic physician in private practice, as well as a speaker known for her witty and engaging style. She has been a natural medicine expert for television, radio and print news outlets and has presented scientific lectures and comedy shows on the topics of health and burnout since 2001. Dr. Loomis's diverse resume includes naturopathic private practice, business consultant, managing editor for the *Naturopathic Doctor News and Review,* departmental director, and instructor of several subjects at the National University of Natural Medicine (NUNM) in Portland, Oregon.

Beth Genly, MSN, now leads the coaching and consulting company, Burnout Solutions (www.Burnout-Solutions.com.) As a speaker and workshop leader, her audiences love her warm, interactive style. After earning her graduate degree in midwifery from Yale University School of Nursing, she worked for 23 years as a nurse-midwife, during which time she taught, provided hands-on care, and worked as a clinical manager. Her midwifery career included working as a clinical provider for the Yale Health Center and a decade serving on the nurse-midwifery faculty at Oregon Health and Science University (OHSU.)

Both authors are available for interviews, keynote addresses and guest speaking opportunities. To contact the authors, please reach out to us on Facebook at www.facebook.com/burnoutsolutions. Or email Beth at beth@burnout-solutions.com.

CPSIA information can be obtained
at www.ICGtesting.com
Printed in the USA
BVHW031212290419
546817BV00001B/60/P

9 780999 137208